Biomicroscopy
for
Contact Lens Practice

© Copyright 1970 by the Professional Press, Inc.

FIRST PRINTING

Library of Congress Catalog Card Number: 68-57482

Published by The Professional Press, Inc.
Five North Wabash Avenue, Chicago, Illinois 60602

Printed in the U.S.A.

Biomicroscopy
for
Contact Lens Practice

by

Joe B. Goldberg, O.D., F.A.A.O.

The Professional Press, Inc.
Chicago

Dedicated to the late
DR. VINCENT J. ELLERBROCK
without whose original encouragement
this book would never have been written,
and to
DR. ALFRED A. ROSENBLOOM, JR.,
whose personal interest and counsel has
made it possible for this book to be
published.

Table of Contents

PREFACE

As the first major publication describing biomicroscopy and its specific use in contact lens practice, this book will be of interest to both the student and the established contact lens fitter.

The development of contact lenses has made it possible for vision to be corrected without using conventional spectacles. Contact lenses are often prescribed to satisfy an individual's cosmetic needs, but they have a particular therapeutic value in the correction of such conditions as aphakia, keratoconus, and keratoplasty, and in low vision. Their psychological importance is seen in their use as cosmetic lenses for blind or scarred eyes.

Although the concepts presented in this book concern both corneal and scleral contact lenses, the primary focus is on corneal lens fitting. Corneal lenses are easier to fit, manage, and control. No other contact lens form has achieved such world-wide success.

Chapter I discusses the role of biomicroscopy in contact lens practice, describes the historical development of the biomicroscope and shows how the principles of biomicroscopy are applied to contact lens fitting. The basic design of the biomicroscope, the phenomenon of reflection as it affects the cornea, and the techniques of biomicroscopic examination are considered in Chapter II. The types of illumination are discussed according to their clinical use and their individual relationships to contact lens practice. Chapter III reviews corneal anatomy and physiology, emphasizing the importance of corneal transparency. The practical application of biomicroscopy is presented in Chapter IV. Its use in the differential diagnosis of the contact lens fit is described, as are the sequential development of corneal pathology induced by contact lens wear, corneal curve and refractive changes found after removal of the lens, and related findings. Chapter V – a conspectus on contact lens fitting – describes how biomicroscopy may be used to determine contact lens modifications. Chapter VI concludes the book with a description of the equipment and techniques of biomicroscopy photography.

In the early years of contact lens development, one could describe contact lens fitting with the maxim, "Caveat emptor!" Today we can proudly exclaim, "Tempora mutantur" (Times are changed). No longer is it necessary to seek contact lens fitting instruction only from private sources, or to rely exclusively on a manufacturer's fitting manuals. The growth and maturity of contact lens practice is reflected in the academic and clinical programs found in all optometry schools, ophthalmological residencies, postgraduate courses sponsored by organized optometric and medical groups, and last, but not least, the various contact lens textbooks now available.

It is my opinion that success in fitting of corneal lenses is directly related to the extent of the practitioner's skill and his knowledge of biomicroscopy as a clinical technique. In preparing this text, I have attempted to distill the knowledge and experience gathered in more than twenty years of service to contact lens patients. It is my earnest hope that the information presented will aid others in contact lens practice.

Joe B. Goldberg, O.D.

ACKNOWLEDGEMENTS

Often, writing a book requires the use of the coordinated skills and knowledge of several people; one person, alone, may find himself traveling a path of exasperation and confusion as he wades through what seems to be an endless amount of material. Although the author must assume the responsibility of the actual writing, others read, criticize and make suggestions.

Therefore, I would like to thank Drs. Neal J. Bailey, John W. Dickerson, Alfred A. Rosenbloom, Jr., Morton D. Sarver, and Bradford W. Wild, for their assistance as technical consultants. My thanks also to Mr. Roy Stealey, for his editorial counsel, and to Mr. Martin Topaz, for his interest and encouragement.

It is also appropriate to express my appreciation to my typists, Mrs. Joan Brandon, Mrs. Edith Jeffers, Mrs. Laura Alman, my editorial consultant; and to Mr. Charles Ericksen, who introduced me to biomicroscopy photography.

I am indebted to thousands of contact lens patients for their unquestioning allegiance during my formative years in contact lens practice, and I thank them for agreeing to sit patiently while I took an unlimited number of biomicroscopic photographs.

Joe B. Goldberg, O.D.

Biomicroscopy
for
Contact Lens Practice

CHAPTER I

Biomicroscopy
and
contact lens practice

Contact lens fitting has made many practitioners aware of biomicroscopy and has given greater emphasis to the need for its use.

Biomicroscopy is the examination of the living eye by means of an instrument which consists of both a controlled illumination source, often called a *slit-lamp,* and a corneal microscope. Biomicroscopy may be considered an intravital, histologic method for the study of the ocular tissues (Berliner, 1949). Today the term, *slit-lamp,* is outmoded, since the slit is only one of the types of diaphragmatic openings available.

Prior to the acceptance of contact lens fitting, the biomicroscope was used only in medical diagnosis. Now, however, it is considered to be a necessary piece of objective instrumentation which is vital to the effectiveness of contact-lens-practice procedures.

When using biomicroscopy for contact lens fitting, one can observe conditions of poor lacrimal interchange, constant bearing areas, epithelial disturbances and areas of incipient vascularization which he may not detect when using lesser degrees of illumination and magnification. Whereas a system of

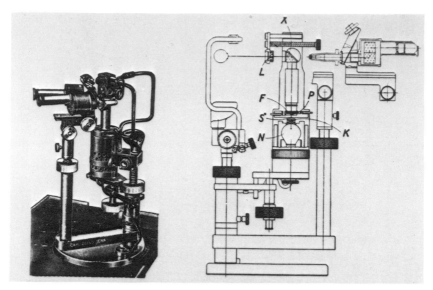

Fig. I-1. Cross section of biomicroscopic equipment (after Comberg). For the sake of clearness the body part of the corneal microscope is shown separately at the right. N, Nitra bulb; K, condenser; S*, slit; P, Rekoss disk with diaphragm; F, Rekoss disk with red absorbing filter and gray glass filter; X, prism; L, illuminating lens. (Courtesy of Carl Zeiss, Inc., West Germany.)

lens-loupe, or any type of objective, high magnification procedures may be used in contact lens practice, there is no system in use today that can equal the effectiveness of the higher magnification and illumination which is provided by the biomicroscope.

The use of the biomicroscope will furnish guidance to the contact lens practitioner concerning the effectiveness of the lens design for his patient and will stimulate him to achieve greater accuracy in creating all contact lens design components. Aided by biomicroscopy, the contact lens practitioner will be more secure in his knowledge that his design will not interfere with the prerequisites for maintaining corneal transparency. The biomicroscope will help the practitioner to decide whether he should change or retain any one or all of the contact lens design components and will facilitate the prescribing of specialized contact lens designs (e.g., small, thin, steep corneal contact lenses; non-circular designs).

Gross, naked-eye surveys of the contact lens fit are not to be eliminated, nor is it suggested that the established black light and fluorescein technique be discarded. Instead, it is suggested that these techniques be classified as additional procedures to be used prior to biomicroscopy.

The biomicroscope is an invaluable ally for pre-contact lens fitting information. It furnishes information which is related to corneal structure

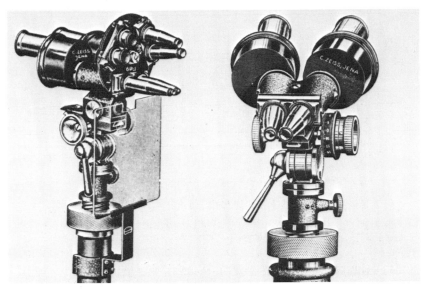

Fig. I-2 (left). Czapski binocular microscope with revolving objectives. (Meesmann, A. Die Mikroskiopie des lebenden Auges an der Gullstrandschen Spaltiampe mit Atlas typischer Befunde. (Courtesy of Urban & Schwarzenberg.)

Fig. I-3 (right). Corneal microscope (Czapski) with Ulbrich drum micrometer for measuring displacement. (Courtesy of Carl Zeiss Inc., West Germany.)

(corneal dystrophy, superficial placement of corneal nerves, quality of conjunctival tissue formations adjacent to the cornea, etc.) which could influence any decision for prescribing contact lenses. In fact, Doggart (1948) stated that only the biomicroscope can detect Fuchs's dystrophy, since this condition involves the disintegration of the endothelial mosaic.

The biomicroscope serves as an excellent guide in all phases of contact lens service – from the period of patient selection through the fitting period, culminating in the individual post-care program. The ability to vary the intensity of illumination and the direction of the beam of light makes this a significant instrument for the evaluation of the cornea during contact lens wear.

When an applanation tonometer is used in conjunction with the biomicroscope, the latter's value is enhanced. Also, one may employ the biomicroscope as a binocular ophthalmoscope for indirect ophthalmoscopy by using (1) a contact lens having a flat anterior surface so that the corneal refraction is eliminated and a virtual image of the fundus is produced in the anterior segment of the eye; (2) a strong concave lens (Hruby lens) which is attached to the instrument and is placed in position directly in front of and a short distance from the cornea so that a focus can be obtained on the fundus; and (3) a strong convex lens placed in front of the cornea to form a real inverted image of the fundus between it and the miscroscope (Duke-Elder, 1962).

5

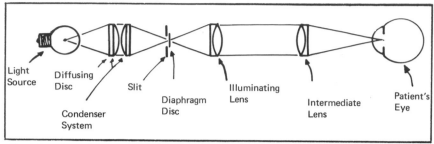

Fig. I-4. Universal slit lamp illumination system. The Parallelepiped created by direct focal illumination with a wide slit.

HISTORICAL DEVELOPMENT OF BIOMICROSCOPY

A knowledge of the development of biomicroscopy will help the student understand the subject's complexities.

In 1891, Aubert presented a binocular corneal microscope at the Ophthalmological Congress in Heidelberg. Czapski (1897) modified the Aubert corneal microscope, and Zeiss added further refinements which made the Czapski-Zeiss corneal microscope better — an erect image with a full stereoscopic effect was obtained by a system of Porro prisms with four reflections; the eyepieces could be adjusted to suit the interpupillary distance of the examiner. However, the value of this microscope was not fully established until Gullstrand (1911) solved the problem of illumination. The design of all subsequent corneal microscopes has been based on these principles.

Prior to Gullstrand's invention, a system of "lens and loupe" was used in which a bi-conex lens formed an oblique beam on the eye from a nearby lamp. H. Wolff first used a carbon filament bulb ophthalmoscope, with light passing through a condensing lens, reflected into the eye by means of an oblique mirror and cast an image of the filament on the retina (Berliner, 1949). This was the first truly focused beam for the examination of ocular tissue.

In 1911, Alvar Gullstrand presented the first rudimentary model of the slit-lamp before the German ophthalmologists in Heidelberg. It was the first time a satisfactory method was made available to examine the anterior parts of the living eye. The Nernst lamp served as the basis for illumination. Its filament was composed of a tightly coiled tungsten spiral, coated with a compound of metallic oxides which became incandescent when electrified. The lamp was rod shaped and therefore suitable for use with a slit diaphragm. Gullstrand developed a method for projecting the image of the Nernst rod in a slit opening to produce a rectangular focal beam. The model of the Nernst slit-lamp illuminating unit constructed in 1908 was used originally to measure the posterior corneal surface. In 1909 it was used in the Uppsala Clinic (Stockholm) as a source of focal illumination for examining the transparent ocular media.

Gullstrand projected the rays of light emanating from an image of the light source rather than those emitted by the luminous body itself, thus making it possible to obtain a controllable beam of strongly focused light without the

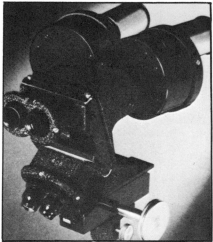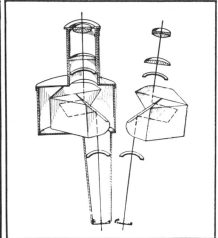

Fig. 1-5 (left). Binocular wide field microscope with Cowan magnification feature; Revolving nosepiece enables quick interchange between low and high powers. (Courtesy of Bausch & Lomb.)
Fig. 1-6 (right). Dissected view of binocular microscope showing arrangement of lenses and prisms. (Courtesy of Bausch & Lomb.)

disadvantage of ordinary oblique illumination.

In 1916 Henker mounted Gullstrand's illuminating system on a horizontal rigid swinging arm in conjunction with the Czapski corneal microscope. This modification permitted relative steadiness as well as mobility so that a more detailed examination of the eye could be made. The light which fell on the part of the eye to be examined was an image of an image. The Nernst filament's image was focused upon the slit, and an image from this slit-enclosed image was in turn directed upon the eye. Both of these images were of uniform light because the filament was homogeneous.

When the Nernst lamp was unavailable after World War I, Gullstrand used the Nitra bulb, which was constructed by winding tungsten in a container filled with nitrogen. Because the Nitra bulb did not furnish uniform light, he made several clinical adjustments in his technique. Vogt made the next major change in the lamp's design by moving the lamp forward so that homogeneous light filled the slit and the illumination was increased. This modification led to the development of the narrow beam of direct illumination (optical section).

Later refinements were made by Koeppe, Koby, Lopez-Lacarrere, Comberg, Arruga, Poser and others.

THE PRINCIPLES OF BIOMICROSCOPY APPLIED
TO CONTACT LENS PRACTICE

Biomicroscopy depends on the full use of focal illumination (light projected by a condensing lens or a series of lenses). At the focal point of such a system the light becomes intensely concentrated. Gullstrand's system, as modified by Vogt,

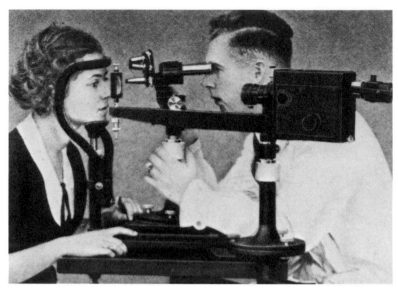

Fig. I-7. Vogt arc lamp. (Courtesy of Carl Zeiss, Inc., West Germany.)

makes it possible to examine the successive layers of the transparent ocular media illuminated by light in exact focus.

The small section of tissues illuminated by the focused light as it passes through the transparent media of the eye corresponds to the size and shape of the beam. There is a marked contrast between the illuminated area and the surrounding area in shadow. This effect, comparable to that of a searchlight beam passing through the sky, is called the *Tyndall phenomenon.* Tyndall used floating dust to reveal the paths of luminous beams through the air (1868). Suspended particles are made visible when one directs an intense beam of light across the field of the objective at angles to the axis of the microscope. Each particle scatters some of this light and the scattered light, which enters the objective from any one particle, is focused as a diffraction disc in the image plane of the microscope ocular, thus becoming visible to the eye by means of increased intensities of light and the apparent increase in size obtained by the formation of diffraction discs.

The cornea, lens, and the vitreous will exhibit the Tyndall phenomenon in varying degrees. It becomes more apparent in pathological conditions.

The normal cornea is avascular, laminated and transparent. The biophysical and biochemical properties of the cornea and the type of insult will determine the nature of corneal reaction. Staining of the pre-corneal film line with fluorescein assists in the exact localization of insult. It also reveals any break which may have occurred on the corneal epithelium. Corneal lesions may or may not be accompanied with vascular invasion. In contact lens practice we are, primarily and immediately, concerned with epithelial staining. Normally, the epithelial surface is protected by the fluid of the precorneal film line. Any condition which prevents normal physiologic passage of fluids or gases through the epithelium causes stasis and resultant epithelial edema.

When the epithelium is abraded, it is loosened. The insult may be superficial, or it may become sub-epithelial. Fluorescein staining may create the impression that the stainable section is larger than it actually is, and attention should be given to the anterior surface of the stained pre-corneal film line since danger arises from possible infection through the exposed corneal section. Hence, an epithelial structural alteration indicates that the controls for the water balance of the cornea and its gaseous exchange are in need of repair.

The biomicroscope becomes a valuable asset in contact lens practice because with it one can observe, objectively, areas of poor contact lens design characteristics (and their immediate effect on the cornea's prerequisites for maintaining transparency) and thus make contact lens design modifications before corneal insult develops to any degree. Thus, one may consider biomicroscopy as an objective control method for observation and the accumulation of data which are related to the effectiveness of a contact lens design.

CHAPTER II

Using
the
biomicroscope

BASIC DESIGN OF THE BIOMICROSCOPE

The biomicroscope is designed for the examination of living tissue. It consists of a binocular microscope mounted on a stand which is used in conjuction with a controlled light source. Its principal parts are (1) an adjustable head rest; (2) a lamp housing suspended on a movable arm which houses an adjustable light source; and (3) a binocular microscope (Fig. II-1).

The modern instruments are used while in parellel focus (referred to as "par-focal alignment"). The stage of the microscope is controlled by a single, raised lever (called "joy-stick" because of its similarity to the control stick used on old-style aircraft) which moves the microscope nearer or farther away, or to either side of the patient. The lamp housing may be moved around its axis through 180° rotation arc. Some instruments have an adjustable prism located at the top of the light. The light source may be controlled for intensity of illumination and any variation of the slit opening. Biomicroscopes have high and low power objective lenses which are attached to the microscope. Additional sets of eyepieces are available for increasing the magnification.

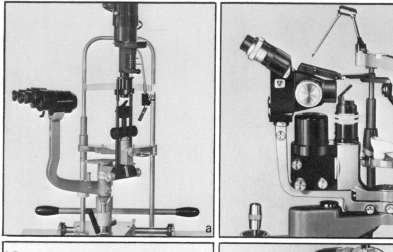

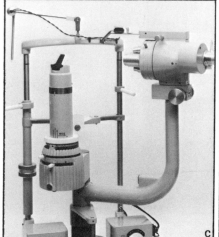

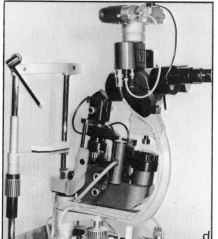

Fig. II-1a. Haag-Streit

Fig. II-1c. Bausch & Lomb, Thorpe

Fig. II-1b. American Optical Co. Campbell

Fig. II-1d. Gambs

The low power objective is used with greater frequency for the initial examination procedures because it has a greater depth of focus and a wider field of vision. High power objectives are used to study the cornea and any irregularities in greater detail. The slit may be adjusted from a thin hairline to a wide, open and round aperture.

The design of the joy-stick biomicroscope makes it possible to use one hand to operate the stage and focus the microscope, while using the other hand to control the angle and width of the incident light. Although it is not my intention to discourage anyone from using a two-position biomicroscope, the newer, par-focal design makes it unnecessary to focus the lamp and the microscope

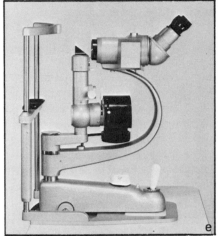

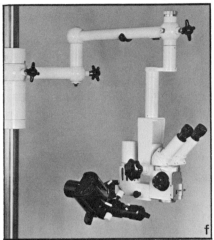

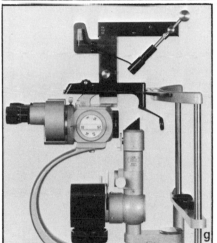

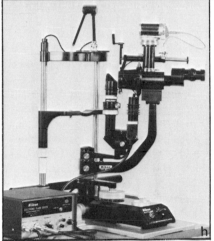

Fig. II-1e. Zeiss Power Zoom
Fig. II-1g. Zeiss, With Hruby Lens and
applanation tonometer

Fig. II-1f. Zeiss Slit-Lamp on Movable
Floor Stand
Fig. II-1h. Nikon

separately, and this makes it easier to learn how to use the instrument. All of the major instruments in use today are excellent for evaluating the contact lens-cornea relationship.

Biomicroscopy should not be used to replace any other system which is used for either gross examination of the eye or examination of the contact lens fit. A conventional lamp that is used for black light and fluorescein examination of the eye should not be discarded. (A black light filter is usually part of a biomicroscope's equipment.) A fluorescein and black light examination is used to assess the characteristics of a contact lens fit for clearance and bearing areas, while the illumination and magnification of a biomicroscope may be used to examine a contact lens fit in greater detail.

THE VARIANT OF CORNEAL APPEARANCE

Koby (1930) presented a fascinating discussion of the phenomena of reflection of light by the ocular media. He stated that the ocular media comprise several *zones of discontinuity* (optical surfaces where the index of refraction suddenly changes). A luminous beam striking such a zone provokes certain optical phenomena, of which reflection is important to biomicroscopy, the others being refraction, polarization, diffraction and fluorescence. One part of the rays is reflected according to the laws of *regular reflection*, the reflected rays being contained in the same plane as the incident, and their respective angles being equal.

The *quantity* of reflected light in biomicroscopy depends chiefly on (1) differences of indices of refraction of the media considered, (2) the degree of polish of the reflecting surface, and (3) the size of the angle of incidence.

Light reflected regularly produces an image of the luminous source at the point of convergence of the rays (real image), or of the prolongation of the rays (virtual image), and observation in the path of regularly reflected rays receives the specular reflection of the surface (its reflex).

One part of the incident light is reflected in a diffuse, irregular fashion and this phenomenon, noticed on the surface of all bodies, makes them visible. Thus biomicroscopy produces the phenomenon of light in the ocular media. The diffuse reflection which occurs at each zone of discontinuity makes it possible to distinguish between the various corneal layers.

The cornea has a complex cellular structure which is heterogenous. (That of glass is homogenous.) The internal dispersion of light caused by the heterogeneity of semi-transparent tissues is known as *relucency*. Therefore, when examined with the biomicroscope, the cornea will vary in appearance according to the type of illumination used. The cornea appears to be transparent when it is examined with diffuse illumination. When the illumination is direct, an opalescent block of light is formed, and the optical effects of the corneal anatomy observed depend upon the transparency of the tissues traversed.

TECHNIQUE OF EXAMINATION

The following directions should be followed in all instances:

1. Lower the room illumination and adjust the instrument to make the patient comfortable.

2. Instruct the patient to place his chin on the chin-rest and forehead against the head-rest, while adjusting the instrument to the proper height.

3. Turn on the instrument and, if a fixation light is used, close the slit diaphragm and instruct the patient to direct his gaze toward the fixation light. If such a light is not used, instruct the patient to direct his gaze toward the examiner's right ear when the right eye is to be examined, and toward the

examiner's left ear when the left eye is to be examined.

    4. Avoid unnecessary illumination.

    5. Issue brief instructions to the patient, to reassure him and to help him relax.

METHODS OF ILLUMINATION

One does not selectively use each method in turn, since, as Doggart (1948a) noted," . . . in actual practice the methods of illumination overlap and swiftly alternate with each other." Clinical procedures for biomicroscopic corneal examination are determined empirically. The order of their use varies, being determined by the individual examiner.

    The principal methods of illumination are:

    1. Sclerotic scatter

    2. Diffuse illumination

    3. Direct illumination

    4. Trans— or retro-illumination

    5. Indirect illumination

    6. Specular reflection

    7. Oscillation

Whereas seven types of illumination are listed, the first six are considered the principal types (although they are not necessarily listed in their order of importance). The seventh, oscillation, serves as an auxiliary function. Thus, seven methods of technique are available for biomicroscopic examination of the anterior segment of the globe, and the efficiency of the instrument in the finer points of diagnosis is related to the selection and application of the proper method of illumination and its control.

    The cornea is observed in optical section according to its histology. The examination should begin with the epithelium and continue with an examination of Bowman's layer, the stroma, Descemet's membrane and the endothelium. Whereas the methods are related for complete corneal examination, as mentioned previously, *there is no established procedure.* Consequently, the types of illumination are described as listed, *for the purpose of suggsting the sequence in a clinical procedure, the order of presentation not indicating their importance.* The author has elected to use *indirect forms* of illumination for an initial corneal survey (since light is not directly on the cornea), and the examination is continued with *direct forms* in the best interests of patient comfort.

Sclerotic Scatter

    This is a special variety of indirect illumination. The light is out of focus on the cornea and the microscope is focused on the cornea (Fig. II-2). An intense beam of light is directed to the sclera near the temporal limbus; the light criss-crosses between the limiting membranes of the cornea and illuminates the circum-corneal region to create a *circum-corneal halo,* which appears as an orange-colored glow around the cornea. Light is reflected backward and forward

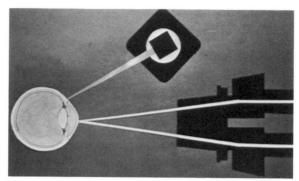

Fig. II-2. Sclerotic scatter. (Photo courtesy Charles Erickson.)

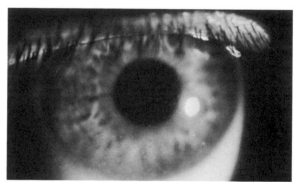

Fig. II-3. Posterior corneal surface precipitates (K.P.). Sclerotic scatter, high magnification.

between the two limiting surfaces of the cornea and is scattered centrifugally around the cornea. Sclerotic scatter exposes areas where the cornea is not transparent. (Fig. II-3).

The procedure is as follows: Narrow the light beam and direct it to the temporal-limbal area of the cornea. Sometimes it is necessary to rotate the prism at the top of the lamp to direct the light. Move the lamp and microscope toward the patient's eye until the light is directed to the proper area. The lamp is usually at an angle of 30 to 60 degrees on the temporal side of the patient's eye, and the examiner may have to change the angle of incident light and coordinate this action with the focus of the microscope on the cornea until the circum-corneal halo is formed. The adjacent area of the cornea is lit because of its own relucency, while a similar glow is observed at other corneal peripheral areas, particularly the side opposite, as the circum-corneal halo is formed.

Sclerotic scatter permits observation of the following:

1. Corneal staining when sodium fluorescein is used. Irregularities will appear as shadows that may be studied in greater detail with other types of illumination (Fig. II-4).

16

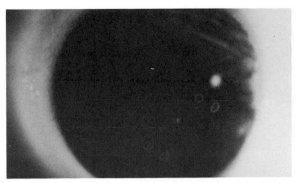

Fig. II-4. Corneal Stippling exposed by sclerotic scatter. Notice circumcorneal halo.

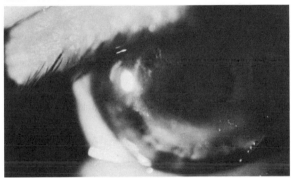

Fig. II-5. Sclerotic scatter exposes bubble formations beneath a contact lens which has been fitted for a corneal graft. The bubbles are under the lens in the para-apical and peripheral areas. The definitions of the graft and surgical scarring are seen.

2. Contact lens scratches. Surface scratches and irregularities of the lenses are exposed. These require further study for detail with other types of illumination.

3. Quality of lacrimal flow when contact lenses are worn. The tears are normally transparent, and the lacrimal flow characteristic is observed only when reference materials, such as lacrimal debris and various particles, are present beneath a lens (Fig. II-5).

4. Interference with corneal metabolism. Because there may be an improper lens-cornea relationship, one may observe epithelial disturbances such as punctate, stippling, epithelial edema, irregular edematous lines epithelial dimpling, or any loss of continuity of the epithelial surface (Figs. II-6,7).

Diffuse Illumination

Incident light, out of focus, is directed to the cornea and provides a general picture of the anterior corneal surface. The iris and limbal areas are illuminated, and obvious corneal changes are revealed. Tinting the tears with sodium

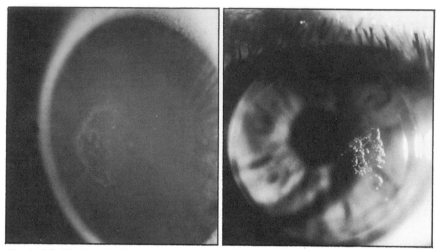

Fig. II-6 (left). Central, circumscribed, corneal edema seen with sclerotic scatter.
Fig. II-7 (right). Foreign material on a contact lens front surface. Sclerotic scatter, low magnification.

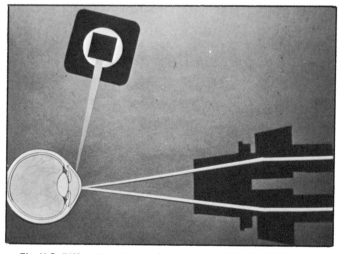

Fig. II-8. Diffuse illumination. (Photo courtesy Charles Erickson.)

fluorescein in this type of examination is a valuable diagnostic aid for contact lens practice. Sodium fluorescein enhances diagnostic procedures when it is used with a cobalt blue filter and biomicroscopy for contact lens practice (Fig. II-8).

With diffuse illumination, low or high magnification, the fit may be examined for the following:

1. Quality of peripheral clearance. Peripheral corneal clearance should be continuous, especially in the superior quadrants. Any discontinuity of peripheral

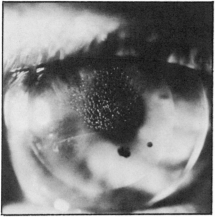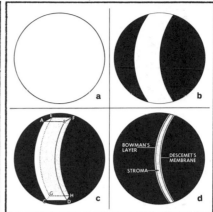

Fig. II-9 (left). Diffuse illumination used to inspect a corneal lens fitted for an aphakic eye. Central zone accummulation of bubble formations, posterior corneal surface pigmentation (the result of pigment migration during surgery, and an outline of the lenticular or optical prescription element, on the front surface of the contact lens).

Fig. II-10 (right). Direct illumination. (a) Diffuse illumination exposes the entire cornea. (b) The peripheral corneal areas become dark when the slit diaphragm is reduced and the illumination is changed to direct illumination, broad beam. Only the anterior corneal surface is exposed at this time. (c) Further reduction of the slit diaphragm removed more light from the peripheral corneal area and the anterior and posterior corneal surfaces are exposed when the illumination is changed to direct illumination, medium beam. ABCD represents the anterior corneal surface; EFGH represents the posterior corneal surface. (d) An optical section is formed by direct illumination, narrow beam (the width of the beam is 1.0 mm or less). The epithelium and endothelium are not exposed in an optical section when the cornea is normal.

clearance indicates corneal bearing, and corneal interference is induced when a corneal lens impinges on the superior limbal areas or encroaches on the superior sclera.

Air bubbles may be forced beneath a lens by the blink when the peripheral curve or curves are too flat (Fig. II-9). The bubbles can stagnate and induce corneal interference. Similarly, when the peripheral curve is too steep, interference with lacrimal interchange is induced, and metabolic waste may not be dissipated beneath the lens properly; gaseous bubbles form in the apical areas and create corneal interference.

2. Quality of apical clearance. When compared with conventional black light-fluorescein examination, the magnification and illumination of a biomicroscope reduces the diagnostic error for the determination of apical clearance. We are able to observe the central dye patterns in greater detail. With diffuse illumination, using low or high magnification, the apical clearance areas will have various hues, according to the degree of clearance, while apical bearing areas will appear dark. Since an alignment fit is basically a *minimal apical clearance fit*, a more expert diagnosis may depend on biomicroscopic examination.

19

The intermediate bearing areas will appear dark. Thus, one may learn to judge how much to reduce an optic zone diameter dimension with this procedure (Fig. II-10).

Peripheral Clearance — Intermediate Zone Bearing — Apical Clearance

The width of intermediate zone bearing, observed with diffuse illumination, may be related to the overall lens size and the known value of the optic zone diameter. In this case, if the optic zone diameter is 7.8 mm. and the overall lens size is 8.8 mm., the width of the intermediate bearing area may be judged to be 0.4 mm. Thus, the optic zone diameter may be reduced 0.8 mm. to form an optic zone diameter of 7.0 mm.

The procedure is as follows: Make the beam 2 mm. wide or wider. Direct incident light to the eye at oblique angles (30 to 50 degrees). Move the microscope toward the patient's eye and focus on the area to be observed. The light illuminates the entire corneal surface, although it is not in focus (Fig. II-11).

Diffuse illumination permits observation of the cornea, sclera, lids and conjunctiva (Figs. II-12,13,14,15,16). It also permits a study of contact lens surface characteristics, lacrimal flow characteristics as indicated by the movement of lacrimal debris and particles beneath a corneal lens, and characteristics of contact lens fit, including scleral encroachment, limbal impingement, corneal bearing areas, quality of peripheral and apical clearance and, generally, the lens position (Fig. II-17).

Direct Illumination

This is the most useful and most frequently employed type of illumination (Doggart, 1948). It is valuable for studying the cornea in detail, the characteristics of a contact lens fit, and corneal effects induced by contact lens design. Doggart (1948b) wrote: "The light is directed obliquely into the eye in a beam, which, intensified by all the advantages of a dark background, illuminate brilliantly the opaque structures, and throws into relief minute optical differences in the transparent media . . . Minute differences in the media are thus made apparent, areas of different refractivity are differentiated, and opacities of a degree so slight as not to be otherwise detectable are rendered visible."

Direct illumination is divided into three classifications: (1) Broad or medium beam; (2) narrow beam, and (3) conical beam. Each classification is designed for a different purpose.

Regardless of the beam used, the light and the microscope are focused at the same point, the optical beam traverses the cornea obliquely, and the following will be observed.

1. The external and internal surfaces appear curved, since the corneal anatomy and the angle of incident light affect the degree of the curvature of the arc.

2. Because there is a loss of intensity of light caused by reflection, dispersion and refraction, it is often necessary to increase the illumination.

20

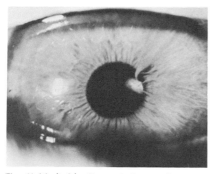
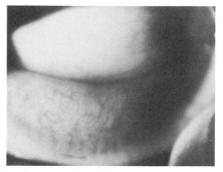

Fig. II-11 (left). Congenital posterior synechia observed with diffuse illumination, high magnification. (This condition does not preclude good contact lens wear.)
Fig. II-12 (right). Palpebral conjunctival injection; diffuse illumination, high magnification.

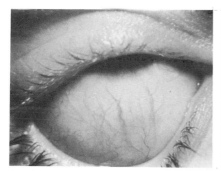
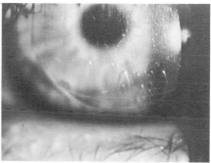

Fig. II-13 (left). The limbus observed with diffuse illumination.
Fig. II-14 (right). Poor wetting of a corneal lens surface. Diffuse illumination, high magnification.

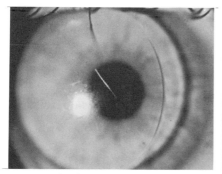
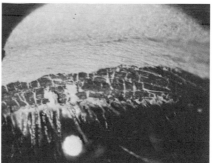

Fig. II-15 (left). A scratch on the front surface of a corneal lens observed with diffuse illumination.
Fig. II-16 (right). Upper lid mascara observed with diffuse illumination, low magnification.

21

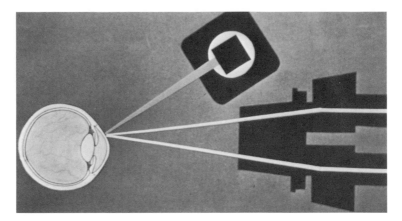

Fig. II-17. Direct illumination. (Photo courtesy Charles Erickson.)

3. An optical section is formed when the width of the slit is reduced; the rectangular block formed is a parallelepiped prism (Figs. II-18,19).

4. The optical density of the medium is caused by the degree of relucency.

Direct illumination with broad beam and medium beam allows one to observe the quality and characteristics of the front surface of the contact lens when it is worn, and to observe the fit in the apical and peripheral areas. The lacrimal flow characteristics may be observed when the incident light is changed to greater than 55 degrees. Bubble formations beneath the lens, as well as superficial epithelial disturbances, may be observed (e.g., punctates, stippling, epithelial indentation, corneal scratches and various forms of corneal abrasions).

The quality of clearance areas may be assessed using direct illumination, medium or narrow beam, low and high magnification; and when the tear layer is stained with fluorescein, white light or a cobalt blue filter may be used. I have found that it is easier to judge the apparent depth of the clearance areas and the quality of the bearing areas when fluorescein is used to stain the tears, although this is not a prerequisite. It is my opinion that the strong illumination of the biomicroscope, not the amount of dye used, stimulates tearing and may temporarily change the quality of the dye pool, giving rise to misleading information about the apparent depth of clearance areas.

When the light and the microscope are focused on the front surface of the dye-stained tear layer, one will see (1) light reflected from the front surface of the contact lens, (2) a dark area which represents the contact lens thickness, (3) the front surface of the dye-stained tear layer. One should traverse the plane of the dye-stained tear layer from one edge of the lens to the other to judge the apparent depth, or quality, of clearance or bearing in any corneal area. Clearance is represented by the full quality of the lacrimal fluid; a reduction of fluid in any area represents less clearance, and corneal bearing appears as a dark, circumscribed area of no fluid.

22

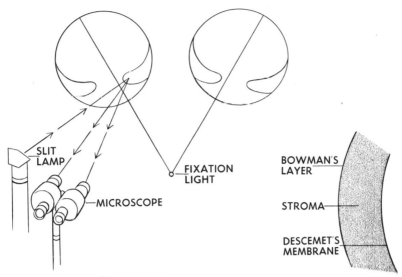

Fig. II-18. Optical section of a normal cornea.

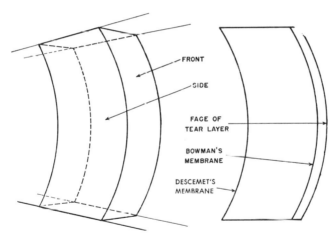

Fig. II-19. Parallelepiped and optical section.

After a corneal lens is removed, the cornea may be examined in greater detail with this type of illumination. This technique is discussed further in Chapter IV (Figs.II-20,21,22).

Procedure for Direct Illumination, Broad Beam

Make the width of the beam 2 mm. or slightly more, and focus the light and the microscope on the same corneal area. Traverse the cornea from the temporal to the nasal limbal areas to examine the cornea (and the contact lens fit). The

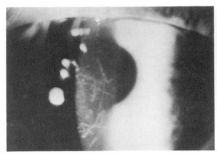 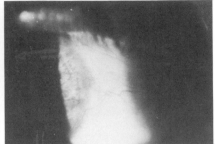

Fig. II-20 (left). Direct illumination, medium width beam. A series of superficial corneal abrasions caused by the movement of a small, foreign particle beneath a corneal lens.
Fig. II-21 (right). Scleral and limbal vessel changes observed with direct illumination, wide beam.

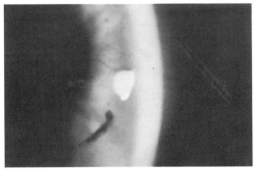

Fig. II-22. Direct illumination, broad beam. Posterior corneal pigmentation in keratoplasty (at 5 o'clock). Remnants of vascularization induced by surgery which remain in the hosts cornea may be seen, faintly, in the middle and upper areas.

anterior corneal surface (and the anterior surface of the contact lens) may be examined. To evaluate the contact lens fit, clearance and bearing areas as well as lacrimal flow characteristics beneath the lens are assessed. An optical section is not formed, and observation is restricted to the areas described above.

Procedure for Direct Illumination, Narrow Beam

A further reduction of the width of the beam of direct illumination forms an optical section, whereby a thin slice of tissue can be thrown into bright contrast with its unilluminated surroundings (Figs. II-23,24,25). The optical section formed is not a frontal view, but a sagittal or coronal view. The optical section has been compared to a knife which cuts the tissue through its entire thickness and exposes its internal features. A thin optical section is important because it affords accurate information for diagnosis and localization of corneal

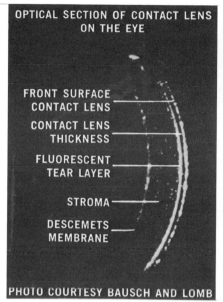
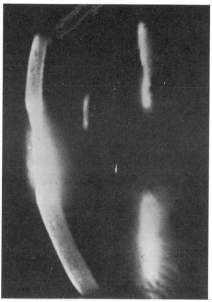

OPTICAL SECTION OF CONTACT LENS
ON THE EYE

FRONT SURFACE
CONTACT LENS

CONTACT LENS
THICKNESS

FLUORESCENT
TEAR LAYER

STROMA

DESCEMETS
MEMBRANE

PHOTO COURTESY BAUSCH AND LOMB

Fig. II-23 (left). Optical section of contact lens on the eye.
Fig. II-24 (right). Keratomycosis. The loss in corneal thickness is clearly visible using direct illumination, narrow beam. (Photo courtesy Carl Zeiss Co., West Germany.)

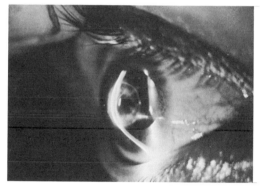

Fig. II-25. Optical section for keratoplasty. (Photo courtesy Carl Zeiss Co., West Germany.)

interference. The optical section (also known as the *parallelepiped of Vogt*) is always bent in the direction of the incident light, and its form varies with the angles of incidence and observation. When the slit is made narrower and the angle of incident light is 25°, or greater, less of the anterior corneal surface is illuminated, and corneal layers appear in section and depth. The optical section

25

becomes a conjunctival prism when it is used to examine the limbal vessels, sclera and conjunctiva.

An optical section is useful and valuable for localization of depth. The stereoscopic image furnished by the microscope allows the relative position of corneal disturbance to be estimated. Superficial epithelial interference (e.g., punctates, epithelial indentation, stippling, foreign bodies, etc.) will have a bright stain, or when fluorescein has not been used, will appear without shadows on the anterior band of the parallelepiped. Objects located in the deeper corneal layers will project shadows, allowing the objects' position to be judged. Posterior corneal disturbances are seen on the posterior band.

The lamp and the microscope may be moved slowly over the cornea until the interference (or object) appears in the optical secton. While this is done, the variations in corneal thickness may be observed.

The technique for identifying the optical section (corneal prism) is as follows:

1. Instill one or two drops of sodium fluorescein into the eye to tint the tears green, for easy identification of the anterior corneal surface.

2. Position the lamp angle between 25 and 35 degrees and open the slit diaphragm to establish diffuse illumination.

3. Slowly reduce the width of the beam to form the optical section.

Direct illumination with broad and narrow beams permits observation of the cornea, lids, conjunctiva, and sclera. It reveals contact lens surface characteristics, bubbles beneath a contact lens, and clearance and bearing areas of a contact lens on the corneal apical and para-apical zones.

Direct illumination with the narrow beam permits determination of the depth of corneal lesions.

Procedure For Direct Illumination, Conical Beam

A small, circular aperture is substituted for the ordinary, or elongated, slit when the vertical height of the slit is reduced and a concentrated pencil of light, similar to that of a searchlight, is formed (Fig. II-26). The angle of incident light is approximately $25°$ to the patient's eye. The light and the microscope are focused on the patient's cornea. The vertical height of the slit is reduced by a lever on the slit-lamp. When the conical beam is formed, move the microscope nearer to the patient's eye and focus the beam in the aqueous. Aqueous particles, if present, may be detected as they float through the conical beam and resemble snowflakes after dark as revealed by a street lamp.

Direct illumination with the conical beam permits observation of advanced turbidity of the aqueous and abnormal opalescence of the anterior chamber.

The slight "flare" revealed by the conical beam is physiological, although stray granules of iris pigment are often found floating in the healthy aqueous. Academically, the conical beam has significance for discovering aqueous disturbances but has little direct relevance to contact lens practice.

According to Doggart (1948b), the following abnormalities of the anterior chamber may be observed with this technique: (1) increased turbidity (flare); (2) abnormal particles — round cells (leukocytes or erythrocytes), crystalline forms

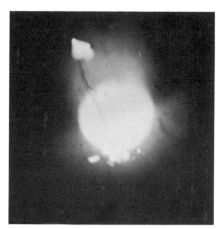

Fig. II-26. Direct illumination, conical beam. Vessel remnant in host cornea in a case of keratoplacty.

(crystals from the lens capsule); (3) heavy fluid accumulations — hyphaema (collection of blood in the anterior chamber), hypopyon (collection of pus in the anterior chamber, consisting mainly of leukocytes entangled in fibrin); (4) larger fragments — flocculent shreds (occur in acute gonococcal iridocyclytis), detached intra-ocular structures (iris pigment which migrates to the aqueous after trauma), foreign bodies (worms, et cetera); (5) vitreous network (tremulous substance entangled in a fine meshwork from subluxation of the lens and after capsulotomy); (6) adventitious reticulation (possible sequel of interstitial keratitis, ruptures of Descemet's membrane, fibrin accumulation upon non-specific kerato-iritis).

Trans-illumination or Retro-illumination

This type of illumination requires the surface of one of the deeper structures to reflect light back toward the cornea. Light can be reflected from the iris or the front surface of the crystalline lens while observation is slightly to the side of the reflected light. Part of the light beam which enters the eye undergoes a change in direction. A portion is absorbed by pigmented screens inside the globe, and another is reflected (producing the red reflex seen in ophthalmoscopy) while the remainder of the beam re-traverses the ocular media (Fig. II-27).

There is usually an overlapping between indirect illumination and retro-illumination. For both types of illumination, the incident light is directed to the iris at an oblique angle and, because the opaque quality of the iris allows it to serve as a reflecting screen, the cornea is illuminated from behind by the reflected light. Indirect illumination (to be discussed later) requires the light to be focused immediately adjacent to the area to be studied. When the microscope is focused on the iris, it is observed in direct illumination; any iritic pathological condition which lies adjacent to the directly illuminated iris portion is, therefore, observed with indirect illumination. The iris cannot be observed with

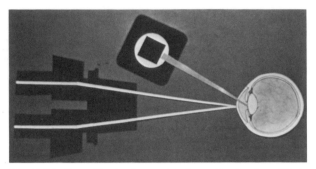

Fig. II-27. Retro-illumination and indirect illumination. (Photo courtesy Charles Erickson.)

retro-illumination.

While retro-illumination is used, part of the cornea will be observed by the retro method and part by the indirect. Conversely, indirect illumination of the cornea is achieved by some of the light reflected from the iris or lens, or both. Because of this overlapping, the practitioner cannot always make a clinical distinction as to which method he is actually using at any given point in the examination.

When a corneal portion is to one side of the beam and some of the light reflected from the iris or lens, or both, illuminates the area of observation, color effects will be created. With retro-illumination, edematous corneal epithelium will have a brownish color when the iris is brown and will appear grey when the iris is of another color. Corneal interference may be observed in the path of reflected light from the iris.

For the procedure of retro-illumination, the beam is between 1.0 mm. and 2.0 mm. wide and is directed to the iris or crystalline lens. The microscope is focused on the cornea and observation is to one side of the beam of incident light. The angle of incident light and the focus of the microscope are changed to study corneal interference. When it is absent, there is no alteration of the normal anatomical corneal structure.

Retro-illumination permits observation of (1) corneal edema (usually of the epithelium, but sometimes of all corneal layers); (2) corneal vascularization; (3) corneal lesions and deposits; (4) deposits on Descemet's membrane; (5) abnormalities of the anterior portion of the crystalline lens (Figs. II-28,29,30).

A corneal disturbance, unique to contact lens practice, is a gray-white, circumscribed area located in the apical zone which usually corresponds to the lens position. It has been named *central corneal clouding* (Korb and Exford, 1968) and *round edema* (Ericksen, 1964 and Girard, Soper and Sampson, 1964).

This gray-white area may be observed silhouetted against the dark pupil background with various forms of biomicroscopic illumination, such as sclerotic scatter, retro-illumination and "split-limbal technique," (Korb and Exford, 1968). Central corneal clouding is more difficult to observe when there is a small pupil diameter because it precludes sufficient background contrast. The contrast

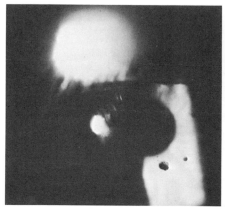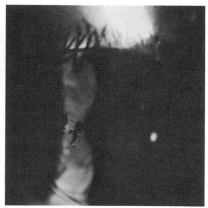

Fig. II-28 (left). Pigment deposits on posterior corneal surface of aphakic patient, retro-illumination.
Fig. II-29 (right). Foreign material on the front surface of a corneal lens seen with retro-illumination, high magnification.

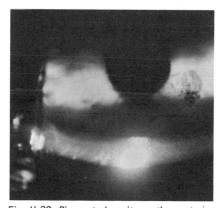

Fig. II-30. Pigment deposits on the posterior corneal surface of an aphakic patient. (The pigment deposits which are seen in light immediately reflected from the iris are exposed by retro-illumination; those on the adjacent, darker areas are seen in indirect illumination.)

between a dark pupil background and the central corneal clouding is enhanced when the pupil is dilated (Sampson, 1967).

While the overall size of the affected corneal area may be related to the overall contact lens size and its optic (central) zone diameter, Korb and Exford reported that the size of the affected area, in itself, is not an indication of the severity of the condition or of the probability of a subsequent abrasion.

Although central circular corneal clouding may be observed with the lens in situ, I prefer to investigate its severity when the lens is removed. Therefore, while the diagnostic biomicroscopic techniques listed above may be used for a *general evaluation* of the severity of the disturbance, *oblique* retro-illumination may be used to examine the corneal apical area in greater detail.

The practitioner should instruct the patient to direct his gaze to the biomicroscope's fixation light which is placed at his eye level. Coordinate the slit-lamp and the microscope in the same plane at 55 to 65 degrees temporally. Move the slit-lamp slowly around an arc which is never more than 10 degrees either nearer to or away from the patient. The position is correct when light reflected from the nasal portions of the iris illuminate the corneal apical area. It may be necessary to move the microscope stage with the joy stick to focus it on the corneal apical area. Because this procedure also moves the slit-lamp and changes the angle of incident light, it is necessary to adjust the angle of incident light to correct for this factor.

The practitioner should also observe the corneal apical area in oblique retro-illumination, high magnification for an assessment of the severity. A mild edematous state appears as a series of wavy lines without form (bedewing). More advanced edema encompasses clusters of microcystic formation and/or irregularly shaped masses without form which may be scattered throughout the anterior corneal area.

Indirect Illumination

Berliner (1949) described indirect illumination as combining some features of sclerotic scatter with some of retro-illumination. Focusing a small beam on translucent tissues (e.g., sclera, iris) adjacent to the area under observation allows one to see corneal features which cannot be observed with direct illumination, as well as edematous areas, deep scleral vessels, iris vessels, hemorrhages in the iris. Thus, indirect illumination permits observation of a part of the cornea while the light is focused on another corneal part which is adjacent to the portion to be observed. Corneal interference is observed when it is *adjacent to the path of reflected light from the iris.*

The incident light beam should be at a wide angle to the axis of observation, and, when the microscope is focused back and forth, the plane of the feature under observation is more easily judged. (Oscillation of the beam permits variable illumination which accentuates certain features perhaps overlooked in fixed illumination.) When using indirect illumination, we inadvertently swing into retro-illumination.

The procedure for indirect illumination is as follows: the beam is opened to a width of approximately 1.0 mm. to 2.0 mm. The angle of incident light is approximately $60°$ to $70°$. The light is directed to the pupil and iris. The microscope is focused on the corneal area to be studied. To observe and study corneal interference, the angle of incident light and the focus of the microscope are changed. The area observed will be adjacent to the light beam and the illuminated area. When a corneal opacity is present, notice the different changes in relief and three dimensional quality (Figs. II-31,32).

Indirect illumination permits observation of corneal lesions, opacities,

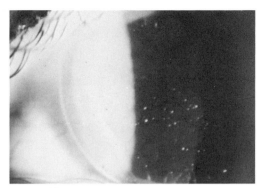

Fig. II-31. Lacrimal debris beneath a corneal lens observed with indirect illumination.

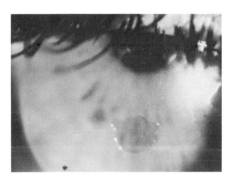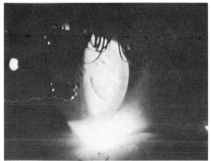

Fig. II-32a (left). Bubble beneath a corneal lens observed using diffuse illumination.
Fig. II-32b (right). Same bubble seen with indirect illumination.

deposits, surface irregularities, and vascularized areas; changes in the integrity of the cornea; areas of corneal edema; corneal nerves (which appear as thin, white lines); wetting characteristics of the contact lens; lacrimal flow beneath the lens and movement of lacrimal debris and particles; bubble retention and dissipation beneath the contact lens. One can also observe the anterior surface of the crystalline lens. (The orange-peel effect observed is called "shagreen".)

When indirect illumination is used and the incident light is directed to the cornea at oblique angles (between 45° and 75°), certain normal conditions as well as those indicating change may be observed. Incident light scattered obliquely through the corneal layers and across the corneal surface is a combination of scatter and indirect illumination. This approach, often called "proximal illumination," is meaningful in contact lens practice when it is used to inspect the limbal areas for old and new vessel formations, the extreme peripheral corneal areas adjacent to the limbus for physiological edema, the superficial and deeper epithelial layers for edema, and the entire field for corneal opacities. Because incident light is reflected from the cornea at various angles, superficial corneal disturbances may be exposed by direct illumination and specular reflection.

The procedure for proximal illumination is as follows: incident light is directed to the cornea at an angle of 45° to 75°, and the microscope is focused on the corneal surface. The angle of incident light is slowly changed by moving the light source toward 65° to 75° and the incident light is directed to the corneal surface. The position of the microscope is changed, as required, to focus on the corneal or limbal areas.

The Zone of Specular Reflection

Doggart (1948), Berliner (1949), and Duke-Elder (1965) have described how a beam of light, when passing from one medium to another, undergoes both transmission and reflection. The amount reflected depends on the difference in refractivity between the two media. This reflection occurs at tissue surfaces, which act as mirrors, so that images are formed of a light source (regular reflection); light is also reflected from irregular, polished surfaces (irregular reflection). The irregular surfaces of the epithelium and endothelium may be considered as an irregular collection of minute concave and convex mirrors whose multiple images are intermingled with the larger single image of the light source seen by an observer looking in the direction of the regular reflected rays, but from the opposite side along a line which forms a similar angle with the normal (Berliner, 1949). The intensity of illumination is very great and may cause patient discomfort.

Goodlaw (1961) commented that specular reflection occurs when the angle of incidence equals the angle of reflection and when the microscope is directed into the reflection.

The procedure is as follows: The beam is opened to a width of 1.0 mm. to 2 mm. The angle of the lamp is set at 45° temporally, and it is moved slowly to the 90° meridian while the microscope is normal to the patient's eye and is focused on the cornea. A catoptric image of the filament is formed on the cornea and is to the right of the incident light beam when the light is incident from the temporal section of the right eye or the nasal section of the left eye. The catoptric image is to the left of the incident light beam when the light is incident from the temporal section of the left eye or the nasal section of the right eye. The microscope is slowly moved nearer to the patient's eye so that the filament of the light is in focus. At this phase of the procedure, the parallelepiped is out of focus. The beam is narrowed and the parallelepiped is slowly moved toward the filament. The microscope is focused and the angle of incident light is changed to expose the posterior corneal surface. (Note: the first mirror reflection observed is from the front surface of the cornea). When the microscope is slowly moved laterally and focused on the posterior corneal surface, suddenly, the classic mosaic pattern of the corneal endothelium will be exposed. The endothelium, which will appear as a fine (web-like) mesh having a yellow-golden glow, is adjacent to the catoptric image of the lamp. The reflected light is very strong and higher magnification should be used for better observation and study. The corneal epithelial surface, as well as the front surface

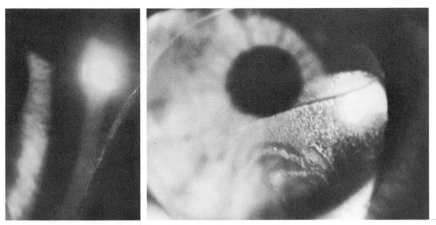

Fig. II-33 (left). Specular reflection. (The image from the posterior corneal surface is seen.)
Fig. II-34 (right). Poor wetting of corneal lens surface. Specular reflection, high magnification.

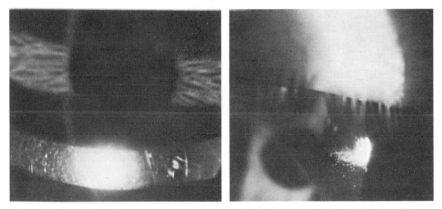

Fig. II-35 (left). Specular reflection exposes scratches on the front surface of a corneal lens, poor wetting characteristics of the front surface of the lens, and mucous formation on the lower part of the lens.
Fig. II-36 (right). Lacrimal debris seen with specular reflection, high magnification.

of a contact lens, is examined in the zone of specular reflection. The areas of the corneal endothelium observed when the incident light is temporally directed are different from those seen with nasally directed light.

Examination in the zone of specular reflection may expose small, posterior surface precipitates. These appear as black dots which mar the endothelial mosaic as do defects in the silvered surface of a mirror (Figs. II-33,34,35,36). This type of illumination is a very delicate method used to observe mucus and cell debris in the tears; to detect and assess changes on the anterior and posterior corneal surfaces; to study the endothelial cells, the anterior and posterior surfaces of the crystalline lens, the shagreen effect, and the epithelial cells of the

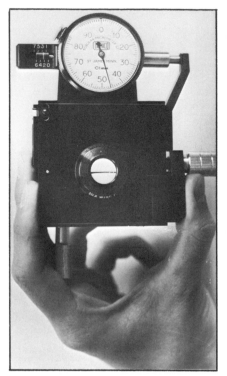

Fig. II-37. Donaldson's Pachometer, used to measure the apparent corneal thickness. (Courtesy Dr. D. D. Donaldson)

capsule. The front surface of the contact lens may be observed during wearing for irregularities such as hairline scratches, surface deposits, and poor wetting.

Oscillation

Koby (1930) stated that one can have the advantage of using several types of illumination successively by displacing the illuminating lens laterally, thus combining direct illumination, retro-illumination, and indirect illumination. The examiner oscillates the light source over an area by moving the beam of light slightly to either side. Slight changes may then become noticeable under the contrasted conditions created by rapid alternation between direct and indirect illumination. Although this technique is a practical blend of all of the methods of illumination previously described, it is the least used of all of the methods of illumination.

The procedure is as follows: for any type of illumination established, the lamp is rotated nearer and farther away from the patient. Using an instrument equipped with a handle which will rotate the light beam 360°, the examiner focuses the lamp and the microscope on the cornea and moves the handle to

34

rotate the light beam. The entire field is observed as the light is rotated, to facilitate further examination of the cornea and thus provide flexibility in technique.

Oscillation permits observation of superficial irregularities in the corneal epithelium, corneal opacities, edematous areas of the epithelium, and small objects or filaments in the aqueous and retrolental space which might be undetected with other forms of illumination.

CORNEAL THICKNESS

With a biomicroscope, one may use a pachometer to measure the apparent corneal thickness (Fig. II-37). Various pachometers are those of Maurice-Giardini, Donaldson and Vickers. Basically, an optical section is formed; the doubling prism mechanism of the pachometer is used to dissociate the image, the front of the rear image is aligned with the rear of the front image, and the measurement obtained is the apparent corneal thickness. While no significant data have been collected or reported correlating this information with the effects on the cornea of lens wear, the availability of pachometers and the awareness of this meaningful procedure may prompt those who fit contact lenses to obtain and record this information as a permanent part of a patient's case history, at the initial, pre-contact lens fitting visit and at all progress fitting and post-care visits. Thus, when they have been related to time, one may be able to correlate changes in corneal curvature and refractive status induced by lens wear with changes in apparent corneal thickness so that he may make effective judgments regarding the etiologic relationships of these changes.

CHAPTER III

Corneal transparency and contact lenses

Besides the obvious necessity for corneal transparency to support the human optical system, the fact that the cornea *is* transparent affords the unique opportunity to observe, with the aid of a biomicroscope, the condition of all the layers of corneal tissue in vivo. Since pathological changes in the various corneal layers (either present before contact lens wear or induced by contact lenses) can affect corneal transparency, it is important that we understand the properties which make the cornea so unique.

Francois and Rabaey (1960) emphasized that corneal transparency is dependent on the microscopic corneal framework and the concentration of histochemical and ultramicroscopic structure. Phase contrast microscopy, historadiography and electron microscopy provide understanding of the inter-relationship of the factors responsible for the maintenance of corneal transparency. Interestingly, a very cloudy cornea sometimes shows only slight histological changes. The "lattice" theory of corneal transparency proposed by Maurice (1962) is based upon the regular arrangement of the corneal fibrillae.

37

The fibrillae are uniform and equal in diameter and are arranged in a regular two-dimensional lattice formation (Davson, 1963). Maurice compared the fibrillae to a diffraction grating where scratches are very close to each other with a spacing less than the wave length of light. Under these conditions there is very little scattering of light, except in the direction of the incident beam, and the cornea will appear transparent. Corneal swelling causes the rows of fibrillae to separate from each other with resultant disorderly arrangement and loss of corneal transparency. A swelling of the mucoid in which the fibrillae are embedded can cause cloudiness by light scatter.

Davson (1963), in discussing corneal transparency, referred to the manner in which light is transmitted by a material rather than its ability to transmit light. Describing the perfect optical image created by dark glasses which may reduce the transmission to ten per cent of the incident intensity, he compared the glasses with an opal screen which may reduce the intensity less, but precludes the formation of an image because of the *scattering* of the light. Davson concluded that the cornea is transparent because less than one per cent of the light is scattered.

Since corneal swelling is associated with a loss of corneal transparency, the design dimensions of the contact lens must not cause it to impinge on an area associated with the oxygen supply requirements for the eye. Metabolic energy is necessary for maintaining corneal thickness and any absence or reduction in the amount of oxygen necessary for supplying this energy will create an increase in corneal thickness and therefore result in fogging of vision (Davson, 1963; Smelser and Ozanics, 1952).

Cogan and Kinsey (1942) suggested that the cornea remains transparent because the limiting layers of the cornea behave as semipermeable membranes and an osmotic difference acting across them counters the swelling pressure of the stroma. This osmotic difference results from the secretion of an aqueous humor hypertonic to blood, and therefore, hypertonic to the stroma which is in equilibrium with the blood.

Disagreeing with this hypothesis, Maurice (1960) commented that the mechanism proposed does not appear to be feasible. He stated that the endothelium is permeable to the important solute of the aqueous humor, and that the cornea apparently is able to maintain the difference in osmotic pressure by the action of its own metabolism. According to Maurice, the epithelium and endothelium, themselves, are barriers to water transfer, and he considered this significant. He stated that the resistance exists only in the epithelium and not in Bowman's layer and that the resistance is probably in the epithelial surface layer since this is very sensitive to the touch. Neither does the resistance present in the endothelium occur in Descemet's membrane.

Adler (1959) described the metabolic activity of the cornea as involving respiration and glycolysis. Respiration, which takes place mainly in the epithelium, requires the presence of oxygen and results in the production of carbon dioxide and water and the liberation of energy. The energy thus liberated is available for cellular activity and for maintenance of tissue temperature.

Glycolysis may take place in either the presence or absence of oxygen and in either the epithelium or the stroma.

The sources of an adequate oxygen supply to the cornea are the pre-corneal fluid, the limbal capillaries, the aqueous humor, the oxygen from the atmosphere. The pre-corneal fluid furnishes oxygen to the cornea and helps carry away metabolic waste materials. A contact lens may reduce and/or obstruct lacrimal flow characteristics in areas of corneal bearing, and may create a decrease in the oxygen supply furnished by both the pre-corneal fluid and the limbal capillaries. As a result, there is (1) an increase in lactic acid, (2) interference with corneal gaseous exchange requirements, and (3) formation of carbon dioxide bubbles underneath the contact lens which cause pressure against the corneal epithelial surface and create restricted local areas of corneal epithelial edema.

When the epithelial surface is no longer a barrier to the invasion of water into the cornea and the contact lens design is not modified in situ, the condition worsens. The edema induced in the epithelium may spread to the deeper corneal layers and cause severe corneal damage.

The epithelium is important for carbohydrate metabolism of the cornea. In the epithelium, glucose is broken down into lactic acid; and, although lactic acid cannot be oxidized further by the stroma, further oxidation can take place in the epithelium, where a complete system exists for the oxidation of glucose into carbon dioxide and water.

Ashton (1960) described the cornea as avascular with sluggish circulation and having minimal oxygen supply. He reported that lactic acid concentration in the cornea becomes lower when the oxygen tension in the tear fluid becomes higher. The cornea produces lactic acid at a high rate whenever the oxygen supply to the cornea becomes insufficient to maintain maximal respiration.

Smelser and Chen (1955) reported that the concentration of lactic acid begins to rise and increases a function of the time during which an improperly fitted contact lens is worn. They found a decrease in corneal transparency coincident with the rise in lactic acid concentration.

Hirano (1959) observed a widening of the intercellular spaces, disarrangement of corneal epithelial cells, thickening of the stroma, dilatation of iris vessels and glycogen changes when an improperly fitted contact lens was worn. These findings show that a proper glycogen reserve must be maintained by providing adequate pre-corneal fluid circulation and by permitting the cornea to adapt slowly to its new environment.

Hill and Fatt (1964a) found that a very secure fitting contact lens creates a rapid decrease in oxygen underneath a contact lens. To demonstrate the need for oxygen underneath a contact lens Smelser (1952) added oxygen to the tear layer to create an oxygen bubble underneath the lens. He observed a gradual reduction of the size of the bubble as the oxygen was used by the cornea.

Clincal experience leads one to recognize that the metabolic processes of the cornea must adapt to the new environment created by a corneal contact lens. Hence, the "adaptive period" for the new contact lens wearer may be considered to be the time required for the histochemical adjustment of the corneal metabolism to the vision aid.

Although a contact lens, by weight, becomes a constant force against the corneal surface, there is little clinical evidence to suggest that it *completely* disturbs the orderly arrangement of the stroma fibrillae or affects the tissue fluid pressure of the cornea.

Adler (1959) stated that the transparency of the cornea becomes temporarily impaired when abnormal pressures are applied to it and he associated any loss of transparency, not only with the imbibition of fluid, but also with physical changes in the stroma, since the cloudiness disappears immediately when the pressure is lowered.

When a contact lens obstructs the cornea's access to oxygen, there is interference with the normal dehydration mechanism and the cornea becomes deturgesced, exhibiting increases in thickness and turbidity, and the lactic acid content increases. Coincident with the increase in lactic acid, there is an increase in the density, thickness, and water content of the cornea.

When a contact lens causes tears to be retained, over the corneal surface, interference with tear evaporation at the surface occurs, and osmotic imbalance may result from either an increase in the salt content of the cornea or a decrease in the salt content of the tears. If one assumes that the imbalance is caused by the former rather than the latter, it should be possible to influence epithelial fluctuations by changing the contact lens design and thereby change the composition of the tears.

STRUCTURE OF THE NORMAL CORNEA

Doggart (1948) pointed out that biomicroscopy has proved that certain congenital abnormalities of the eye are more common than has generally been supposed, and while they are found in as many as 50 per cent of the people examined, many of these abnormalities are trivial, require no treatment, and do not appreciably impair the function of the eye; the main concern of the patient and examiner is to know whether the condition is stationary or progressive. Doggart (1948) stated that limbal vessels, conjunctival vessels, and the corneal nerves may vary in appearance in different patients so that a normal cornea may have several forms.

A preliminary survey of the cornea with the biomicroscope is made with sclerotic scatter, diffuse illumination, retro-illumination, indirect illumination and the broad beam of direct illumination. The cornea is examined in depth for separate layers with the narrow beam of direct illumination (optical section).

Berens and Zuckerman (1946) suggested that the practitioner first examine the cornea as a whole, noting its size, thickness, peripheral rings of opacification, transition area at the limbus; and then observe the cornea in detail.

Francois and Rabaey (1960) stated that the transparency or opacity of a tissue is determined by its structural frame and by the presence and concentration of certain substances. They used modern instrumentation and

40

techniques (phase-contrast microscopy, historadiography, and electron microscopic examinations) to describe corneal anatomy.

Epithelium

The epithelium consists of five cellular layers and is from 50 to 100 microns thick. The characteristics of the *basal cells* are as follows: they rest on Bowman's layer; are cylindrical, squat, or elongated; have an ellipsoid nucleous; contain nucleic acid, desoxyribonucleic acid in the nucleus, and ribonucleic acid in the cytoplasm.

The cells of the deepest row are dimpled cells, while the cells of the middle layer are irregularly polyhedral. The superficial cells are flat, retain their nucleus, and show no keratinization.

The human epithelium contains glycogen, which is a source of energy. Small granules, homogeneously spread, are found at the basal pole of the cell, which has been reported difficult to see even with great magnification. Francois and Rabaey (1960) considered this to indicate the existence of a strong bond between the polysaccharide and other tissue elements

The corneal epithelium is rich in enzymes. The superficial layers contain less water and have a chemical composition different from that of the other layers. The intercellular substance is a delicate cellular framework which delimits the cells of all parts and is found in the superficial and intermediary layers.

Phase contrast microscopy, which permits the examination of epithelial cells in vivo, show them to have a homogeneous nucleus with nucleoli; and the cytoplasm to contain numerous granules which vary in arrangement in the cells of the different layers.

Electron microscopic examination indicates that the epithelial cell wall is very irregular, especially in the basal and middle layers. The epithelial cells are surrounded by a membrane of irregular thickness. The cytoplasm is denser in the pseudopods and shows a network in which inclusions and granules are visible. The superficial cells show no vacuoles.

The epithelium may be examined with the biomicroscope with diffuse illumination, direct illumination, indirect illumination, retro-illumination and sclerotic scatter (not necessarily in this order). When the narrow beam of direct illumination is sharply focused on the anterior surface of the cornea, the anterior band is doubled and the second band to appear is very homogeneous and represents Bowman's layer. The space between the two corresponds to the epithelium, and purely epithelial changes are confined to this space.

With the narrow beam of direct illumination (optical section), the arc of the section always faces the direction of incident light, and the epithelium is usually assumed to coincide with the anterior band. Doggart (1946) described a variable epithelial edema on the limbal areas, which he believed is not necessarily an unfavorable sign. This condition is known as physiological bedewing of the epithelium ("bedewing" simply indicating a mild degree of edema which may be likened to the fine sprinkling of dewdrops upon a lawn early in the morning) and is observed with indirect or retro-illumination. Apart from the normal peripheral

41

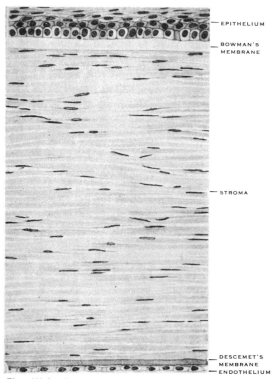

— EPITHELIUM

— BOWMAN'S MEMBRANE

— STROMA

— DESCEMET'S MEMBRANE
— ENDOTHELIUM

Fig. III-1. Cross section of cornea (reprinted from Wolff's Anatomy of The Eye and Orbit published by Blakiston Co.).

bedewing, the normal epithelium has no special characteristics when it is examined with the biomicroscope.

The basal membrane is a fine membrane which lies beneath the epithelial cells and supports them. Under the phase microscope, it appears as a vividly red, thin margin that is continuous (La Tessa et al., 1954; Calmettes et al., 1956). It is thicker at the periphery, where its fibrillar structure is more evident. It contains no glycogen and is not chromotropic. La Tessa et al. (1954) reported that the basal membrane contains plasmogen, which favors adhesion to the epithelial cells.

Bowman's Layer

Historadiographic examination demonstrates this layer as a very fine, dense line underneath the basal cells and a less dense zone near the stroma. Electron microscopy has exposed a mosaic structure created by implantation of basal epithelial cells.

Francois and Rabaey (1960) observed two zones: a dense band measuring 0.5 micron immediately below the epithelium and then a less dense band. The anterior surface is irregular and has crests which protrude among the basal cells. The posterior surface is not sharply circumscribed, and its fibers are continuous with the stroma fibers.

Jakus (1964) considered Bowman's layer to be a modification of the stroma instead of a structureless membrane which contains irregularly oriented fibrils, similar to those contained within the lamellae of the stroma.

Seen through a biomicroscope, Bowman's layer is clearly defined by its thin, white line and is observed between the epithelial layer and the stroma, with the narrow beam of direct illumination in an optical section.

Stroma (Substantia Propia)

The stroma is the thickest layer of the cornea, occupying 90 per cent of its entire thickness. With the biomicroscope it is seen to be non-vascular (except at its extreme edge), having an irregular, granular appearance and an iridescent glow when observed in optical section. The stroma is composed largely of water and collagen fibrils. The remaining solid material, comprising 0.15 per cent of the total, contains lipids, water-soluble extractives and some proteins insoluble in water, and the mucoid substance, which has been identified as mucopolysaccharide (Thomas, 1955).

The structure of the stroma is studied in the optical section or, if the beam is broad, on the lateral surface of the parallelepiped nearest the observer. Koby (1930a) wrote that "the stroma has a fairly regular marbled appearance which is due to the presence of small areas, *arachnoid corpuscles,* which are possibly identical with the fixed cells of the cornea. They appear to be connected both sagitally and frontally. The lamellar structure of the cornea seen in histological examination does not appear in the examination of the living eye and is probably an artifact caused by the reagents."

Electron microscopy has shown that the sclera has thick collagen fibrils which vary in size, while the stromal fibrillae are delicate, identical and have a uniform diameter. The corneal fibrillae are "dirty" as compared with the fibrils of the sclera, and usually stick together in a mass as if they were enveloped by an amorphous substance formed by the fibrillae which covers the meshes. This amorphous substance is the mucoid.

The corneal mucoid appears to be responsible for the stromal property of rapid absorption of water from the environment. This property is of great importance in the maintenance of corneal transparency (Francois and Rabaey, 1960). Transparency is normally assured as long as a certain equilibrium in hydration is maintained; increased water absorption immediately creates a loss of transparency. In a normal cornea, the compact mass of the fine fibrillae and mucoid creates an almost impossible barrier. A historadiographic examination shows the regular arrangement of the fibers parallel to the surface.

When Francois and Rabaey (1960) examined the stroma after swelling, they found that the fibrillae were not thickened and that their structure was less serrated and slack. In their opinion, this finding supports the hypothesis that corneal swelling takes place exclusively in the inter-fibrillar mucoid.

Duke-Elder (1962) stated that in inflammatory conditions, the cornea thickens and the stroma suffers a loss of transparency and appears milky white. Infiltrations and thickenings, localized, diffuse or disciform, can be delineated and fine opacities observed.

DESCEMET'S MEMBRANE

This corneal layer has a thickness of 6 microns and, on routine histological or phase contrast microscopy, appears to have no structure. Baud and Balavoine (1953) described Descemet's membrane as consisting of superimposed lamellae, parallel with the surface. Electron microscopic examination shows a granulated, undulated structure with surface irregularities measuring 0.05 to 0.10 microns.

In a biomicroscopic optical section, Descemet's membrane appears as a thin, narrow grey line immediately posterior to the stroma. In pathological conditions it is frequently folded, indicating the involvement of the deep layers after either inflammation or trauma; the folding (wavy appearance) usually occurs in conditions of hypotony. This layer can separate from the stroma or reduplicate itself after surgery.

ENDOTHELIUM

This single layer of flat cells has no special features. Phase contrast microscopy shows these cells to be suspended in aqueous humor. Their nuclei contains two nucleoli and the cell wall is clearly visible. The cytoplasm shows a large number of granulations, varying in volume, which indicates a very intensive cellular activity.

Jakus (1956) after investigations with the electron micrograph, reported that the endothelial cytoplasm comprises numerous inclusions and infolded membranes. Francois and Rabaey (1960), commenting that these osmophilic infolded membranes, or B-cytomembranes, are present where water transport is very active, concluded that these cells are actively involved in the transfer of water between the anterior chamber and the cornea.

The endothelium is not visible with biomicroscopic optical section. However, small sections may be observed in the zone of specular reflection. Doggart (1948) described the endothelial cells as having well-defined outlines which appear dark, with their shape usually hexagonal, sometimes pentagonal, and occasionally square; the cell layer having a honeycombed appearance. According to Doggart (1948), the endothelium near the limbus appears as if it were interrupted by a series of punched out holes which are caused by localized, backward extensions of Descemet's membrane, named Hassal-Henle warts. These are found especially in adults and the elderly.

LIMBAL AREA

Koby (1930) described this area as less well-defined when observed with a biomicroscope than with the naked eye. Whitish radial fibrous tracts arising from the sclera encroach upon the cornea and occupy a peripheral zone (palisade zone). The vessels form a fine, freely anastomosing network at the limbus and, in the palisade zone, the vessels have a radial distribution and their fine anastomoses extend in fairly regular arcades to the edge of this zone.

With the biomicroscopic techniques of indirect and retro-illumination, the lamp being placed at a severely acute angle (65° to 80°), physiological edema of the cornea is found at the extreme peripheral corneal areas. The edema may be observed with both low and high magnification. Since the limbal palisades may be seen with high magnification, the extent and characteristics of the limbal vessels should be studied so that in contact lens practice, a pre-fitting corneal examination of their appearance may be recorded for future reference.

With diffuse illumination one may observe how scleral vessels extend to the limbus and encroach on the outer corneal peripheral areas. In some patients the limbal palisades are well defined, while in others the areas of physiological edema may obscure limbal definition so that, with diffuse illumination and/or direct illumination, broad beam, one may observe a 1.0 mm. to 2.0 mm. wide grey area between the sclera and cornea.

When using biomicroscopy to examine the limbus, one may expect to find wide variations; these conditions are normal for individual patients. For contact lens practice, it is important to record the appearance of limbal palisades and their extension on the cornea.

CORNEAL NERVE FILAMENTS

In 1830, Schlemm first described corneal nerves, and in 1837 Bochdaalek confirmed Schlemm's report that the corneal nerves originated in the ciliary nerves, consisting of deep and superficial branches which terminate on the corneal surface (Thomas, 1955).

The corneal nerves form an annular plexus at the limbus, usually in the posterior two-thirds, so that the larger nerve fibers are in the deeper layers and the finer filaments are nearer the anterior surface. Nerve filaments have a silky appearance and look like strands. The corneal nerves pass into the stroma in the deeper layers, lose their myelin sheaths within the first millimeter, and branch dichotomously, with an angle of 30° to 60° between themselves, the branches usually having unequal lengths. (Trichotomous branching is sometimes seen, as well as further branch subdivisions.) The branches then form networks at three levels: (1) one within the stroma, (2) one under Bowman's layer, and (3) one within the epithelium. There are no specialized end organs. Rodger, who studied the so-called free nerve endings in the epithelium, found that these endings were not within the epithelial cells, but on and between them and that, in some instances, they reached the surface to form long arcades immediately below the outermost layer of the stratified squamous epithelium (Thomas, 1955).

Corneal nerves are best seen with an optical section and the incident light at a wide angle (45° to 70°). Their courses can be examined when the light beam is focused on them (although the surrounding areas are out of focus). Berliner

45

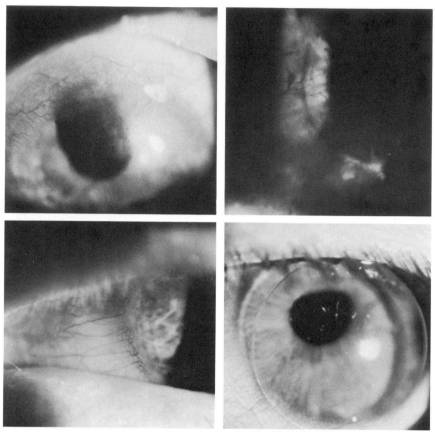

Fig. III-2(a) (upper left). Corneal vascularization (pannus) in the superior corneal quadrants and corneal dystrophy over the nasal pupil area, the result of a healed corneal ulcer. The long, oval pupil shape is the result of cataract surgery.

Fig. III-2(b) (upper right). Corneal vascularization primarily in the hosts cornea which developed after a corneal graft. Branches extend and encroach on the donor's cornea.

Fig. III-2(c) (lower left). Scleral vessel engorgement and proliferation of vessels to peripheral corneal areas induced by an improper corneal lens fit.

Fig. III-2(d) (lower right). Conjunctival injection and limbal vessel proliferation induced by an Astro-Con-2 corneal lens which is fitted flat and with excessive displacement by the blink.

(1949) stated that the number of corneal nerves may be between thirty and fifty.

In the limbal areas, the corneal nerves may enter the cornea in radial directions so that they resemble "spear-like projections" under indirect illumination (Berliner, 1949). The courses of corneal nerves may be followed better with high magnification. While it is rather easy to observe corneal nerves which are nearer the anterior part of the cornea, they appear to lose their definition and end abruptly when their course is traced to the deeper corneal layers, where they terminate.

The corneal nerves become more visible when inflammatory corneal lesions are present which may cause fine sleevelike infiltrates to surround the nerves (Berliner, 1949). However, a loss of normal corneal transparency also occurs, interfering with this increased visibility.

CORNEAL SENSITIVITY

A distinction may be made between *corneal sensibility* and *corneal sensitivity,* since the former describes the cornea's ability to feel or perceive a stimulus to its surface, while the latter describes the cornea's ability to transmit a sensation and respond to it.

The cornea is known to have free nerve endings on its surface. Touch receptors are present, but no heat receptors. The cornea has a highly developed sensitivity for only superficial pain, and large variations in individual response can be found. A decrease in corneal sensitivity from the central areas to the periphery is noticed, with highest sensitivity found in a circular zone immediately surrounding the center of the cornea. Painful sensitivity corresponds to the distribution of nerves because there is a rich supply of free nerve endings in the central corneal areas. Pain caused by corneal irritation is felt as a "foreign body sensation." While receptors for heat and pain caused by heat are absent, there are receptors present for touch, pressure, and pain, their response depending upon the intensity of the stimulus. Cold receptors lie at a deeper level than the free nerve endings and give rise to painful sensations. Also, the sensation of cold is more resistant to anesthesia than is the sense of pain. Although heat receptors are absent, pain stimuli can induce a subjective feeling of heat. Corneal stimuli are conducted to the central nervous system by the ophthalmic division of the fifth cranial nerve.

Photophobia, or pain induced by exposure to light, is believed due to referred pain which results from the close association of the fifth nerve to the optic nerve. This relationship is demonstrated when the condition is relieved by topical anesthesia.

According to Tagawa (1955), the water content of the epithelium apparently is regulated by the nerves. He reported that the amount of water in the epithelial cells was increased after irritation of the trigeminal nerve, so that (after section of the trigeminal nerve) the epithelium became edematous and islands of cells were desquamated, leaving pits in the corneal surface.

Various methods used to test corneal sensitivity rely upon the application of adjustable nylon threads, hairs, etc., to touch the cornea in different areas. Mandell (1965) commented that testing with a battery of hairs of different values is impractical since the hairs can change with the moisture of the surrounding atmosphere. The length and the bend of the filaments are altered while the pressure application is continued until there is a threshold of sensation. These devices, known as "corneal aesthesiometers," "corneal sensibilometer," et cetera, have been introduced by Boberg-Ans (1955), Schirmer and Mellor (1961), and von Frey (1955). Their use in contact lens practice has been

47

described by Strughold (1953) and others.

A Cochet and Bonnet aesthesiometer may be used for routine measurements of the corneal sensation. It is used to test the sensitivity of the upper lid in the center of the tarsal conjunctiva, near the lid margin on its conjunctival surface, and on the peripheral corneal areas to the edge of the pupil before and after adaptation to a daily contact lens wearing schedule.

Schirmer (1963), Koetting (1965), and Kraar and Cummings (1965) have reported on the use of an aesthesiometer to measure corneal sensitivity prior to the fitting of contact lenses. Significant differences in corneal sensitivity may be found among control groups tested with an aesthesiometer. Schirmer (1963) reported that those with lower sensitivities adjusted better to contact lenses. However, these conclusions have not been correlated with contact lens fitting procedures for general acceptance. While some patients exhibit a more sensitive reaction to contact lenses than others, a poor initial response to contact lenses may have a psychological basis.

Stating that wide fluctuations in corneal sensitivity exist between patients, Bier (1966) considered it preferable to make individual tests for corneal sensitivity prior to fitting contact lenses. Success in wearing contact lenses depends upon a multitude of factors, and the results of corneal sensitivity studies are far from conclusive. Information about corneal sensitivity may, in the future, prove of considerable value in the prognosis of successful wearing of contact lenses; but, from our present knowledge, corneal hypersensitivity cannot be considered a definite contraindication to the fitting of contact lenses. In fact, a contact lens patient with reduced corneal sensitivity may need closer observation than the normal patient to make certain that abrasions undetected by the patient do not occur.

Bier (1957) and Dixon (1964) have reported that the sensitivity of the cornea to touch is decreased in patients who habitually wear contact lenses. Corneal sensitivity decreases with age. It is diminished after the age of 45, and a person 60 years old has about half the corneal sensitivity of a person under 20. Corneal sensitivity is also reduced by surgical interference and old scars. However, contact lens patients regain corneal sensitivity shortly after removing the lenses, and recovery may vary among all-day wearers.

When the patient first wears contact lenses, he is immediately aware of a foreign-body sensation with lacrimation and epiphora. As the patient builds up wearing time, he "adapts" to the lenses and no longer feels this sensation. There is a gradual reduction of corneal and lid sensitivity as adaptation to contact lens wear increases. Dixon (1964) commented that this is consistent with the findings of Adrian and Zotterman. They reported that a steady stimulus caused a rapid decline in the rhythm of a sensory nerve impulse and postulated that this decline might be due to a decrease in the excitability of the end-organs or to a gradual increase in their refractory period, or both.

This reduction in corneal sensitivity among contact lens wearers which may cause them to be unaware of corneal involvement during lens wear emphasizes the need for periodic examinations with the biomicroscope. Aphakic patients, as well as others who have reduced corneal sensitivity, may experience minor superficial epithelial abrasions when inserting contact lenses, and be unaware of them.

CORNEAL TEMPERATURES

Corneal temperatures are relatively low when compared to those of the body or other parts of the eye. The lowest temperature is at the corneal apex ($92°$F), while the limbus is normally warmer because of its greater vascularity; the highest temperature is found beneath the upper lid (Mandell, 1965).

While it is doubtful that temperature receptors are present in the cornea, it was found that, in rabbits fitted with scleral and corneal lenses, the corneal temperature increased initially $6°$F, decreased after two or three minutes of lens wear, and became stabilized at approximately the same temperature found during the examination before fitting. Yet, the temperature increased during eye closure (blink or forced blink) while the animals wore the contact lens, and these results were found to be essentially duplicated in humans fitted with scleral lenses (Hill and Leighton, 1963, 1964, 1965a, 1965b).

While authorities agree that there are no corneal heat receptors, contact lens patients report subjective symptoms of burning and stinging which would appear to be related to the presence of temperature receptors.

According to the work of Hill and Fatt (1964), contact lens wear has little effect on corneal temperatures when the eyelids are open and the patient's gaze is in the primary position. Corneal temperature apparently increases when the patient blinks, or when fixation changes reduce the vertical dimensions of the palpebral fissure. It would seem, therefore, that the fitting of corneal lenses within the palpebral fissure, resulting in their minimum movement or displacement in blinking, may actually provide the most compatible physiological lens-cornea relationship.

CORNEAL EPITHELIAL TURNOVER

In early studies, the corneal epithelium was described as being a relatively thin tissue six to eight cells deep of stratified squamous epithelium, the deepest cells being elongated or columnar, the middle cells polyhedral, and the superficial cells somewhat flattened. It was assumed that each layer undergoes cell regeneration separately (Jordan, 1937).

In 1960, Hanna and O'Brien used tritium-labeled thymidine as a cell marker. This was incorporated into the cell nucleus during the premitotic phase to become stable during the remainder of the cell's existence and permitted study of the proliferation and subsequent function of the epithelial cells of the cornea. Thymidine was injected into the anterior chamber of rats' eyes, and the eyes were enucleated at hourly intervals to be studied for the extent of labeling. The amount of tritium-labeled thymidine incorporated in the cells diminished in about four hours, and the degree of labeling became lighter. It was thus possible to distinguish between recently labeled cells and associated migration. The basal cells migrated forward and reached the superficial layers in an average of three days. Although some of the cells sloughed off within three days, there was a complete turnover of cells within seven days. This proliferating activity, plus limiting dimensions of the corneal epithelium layer thickness, caused the cell structure to become more compressed as the cells approached the outer layers of the cornea.

Contact lens wear requires the cornea to support a constant mass which remains in position (14-16 hours average for all-day wearers) while new basal cells are formed in this environment. However, as yet no report has described how this factor influences changes in the basal cell structure of the corneal epithelium over a period of time.

CORNEAL VASCULARIZATION

Corneal vascularization is a symptom of an inflammatory disturbance and will occur when the cornea loses its tissue compactness. Although the condition is readily cured and the cornea appears normal, the vessel walls never disappear.

The cornea is normally avascular and derives its nutrition from the pericorneal vessels. In inflammatory conditions, the cornea obtains additional blood supply from (1) pericorneal congestion or injection of the normal limbal vessels, and (2) formation of new vessels (neoformations), which occur and vascularize the cornea.

Dixon (1964) described the development of corneal vascularization among animals fitted experimentally with scleral contact lenses, while Lauber (1929), Strebel (1937), Delgado (Dixon, 1964) and co-workers reported corneal vascularization induced in human subjects by contact lenses. All observers reported that after wearing was discontinued the blood disappeared from the vessels.

Ashton (1960) showed that a zone of corneal swelling extending to the limbus is essential to the development of vascularization. Cogan and Kinsey (1942) suggested that corneal edema is an important factor if it is prolonged and involves an area near the limbal vessels. A limbal obstruction capable of reducing corneal tissue compactness can cause corneal edema and vascularization.

In corneal lens patients, vascularization is usually caused by overfilling of the limbal vessels. Occasionally, the vessels proliferate a short distance into the clear cornea.

The cornea does not become vascularized when a contact lens induces epithelial trauma because the cornea does not lose its tissue compactness. However, neglect and poor clinical management of a contact lens fit may cause loss in compactness, with resultant stromal edema and vascularization. Biomicroscopy photography may be used to record the appearance of limbal vessels prior to the fitting of contact lenses and throughout all after-care periods.

A distinction should be made between the corneal vascularization which occurs in general pathological conditions (that is, the presence of new vessels filled with blood in the stroma) and the appearance of new vessels filled with blood on the superficial epithelial surfaces in the limbal areas in contact lens wearers. Johnson and Erkhardt (1940) explained the proliferation of capillaries from the limbus into the cornea as an attempt by the latter to bring oxygen to its cells in response to corneal asphyxia. One might question the continued use of the term, *corneal vascularization,* to describe the condition in which limbal vessels overfill and proliferate for short distances into the clear peripheral corneal areas of some contact lens wearers. Instead, we might consider using the term, *limbal vessel proliferation,* for the purpose of clarity and distinctive reference.

Since a variable degree of physiological edema exists in the limbal, or outer peripheral corneal areas, one may expect to find a high incidence of limbal vascular changes when contact lens peripheral dimensions and the position of the lens on the cornea cause asphyxia. Similarly, since the quality of tissue compactness at the limbal areas varies, an improperly designed corneal lens may induce trauma and limbal vessel proliferation.

COMMENTARY

Contact lenses are foreign bodies which may produce corneal physiological changes by causing trauma, by altering corneal metabolism, and by changing the levels of sensation and oxygen tension. These possibilities are eliminated when contact lens design variables are compatible with all of the factors which are related to the maintenance of corneal transparency.

Only a small amount of the cornea is exposed to atmospheric oxygen when it is covered with a contact lens; the amount of exposure is related to the overall lens size and the lid opening. Contact lens wear so reduces the amount of atmospheric oxygen supplied to the cornea that oxygen tension behind a contact lens is below that of atmospheric partial pressure(155 mm. hg.) and the amount of dissolved oxygen in the cornea decreases (Ruben, 1967). Although the deeper layers of the corneal epithelium have a lower oxygen tension, and the superficial epithelial layers use almost all of the available oxygen for their aerobic metabolism, the deeper epithelial layers can obtain oxygen by diffusion from the uncovered areas or from the aqueous humor when the oxygen tension is low at the epithelial side (as when the lids are closed). While the epithelium may experience various degrees of oxygen deprivation during contact lens wear, sustained damage may be precluded by the rapid rate of epithelial regeneration.

The cornea adapts to oxygen deprivation by some unknown mechanism or by use of alternate pathway (e.g., the reduction branch of the glycolytic pathway) that requires less oxygen from the atmosphere to maintain the metabolic processes responsible for corneal transparency (Farris, et. al., 1967). When the lens design is improper or the wearing time is not compatible with the adaptation rate, pathological conditions such as edema, abrasions, pain or vascularization result. It has been suggested that during wearing periods, when the amount of dissolved oxygen in the cornea decreases, prolonged oxygen tension changes may possibly affect corneal contour (Ruben, 1967). After contact lens removal, the cornea readapts to the increased oxygen supply, and returns to pre-wear levels of metabolic function.

51

APPENDIX A

Color plates relating to various types of illumination in Chapter II

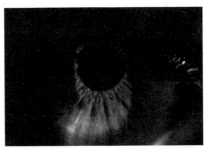

Fig. A-1. The variant of corneal appearance.

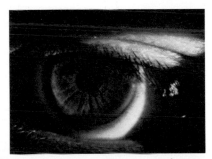

Fig. A-2. Sclerotic scatter: normal cornea.

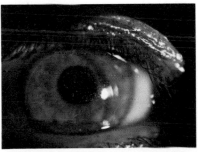

Fig. A-3. Sclerotic scatter: lipid deposits in the tears.

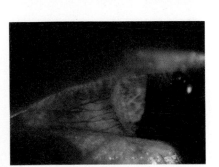

Fig. A-4. Diffuse illumination: scleral vessel injection.

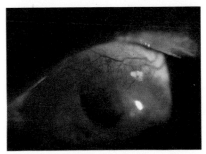

Fig. A-5. Diffuse illumination: pannus, corneal scarring, corneal dystrophy and aphakia.

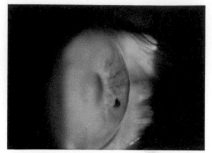

Fig. A-6. Diffuse illumination: lamellar keratoplasty.

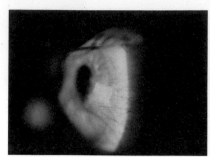

Fig. A-7. Direct illumination (broad beam): pterygium.

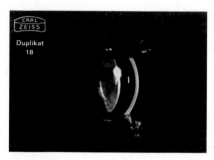

Fig. A-8. Direct illumination (narrow beam): optical section (Photo courtesy Carl Zeiss Inc.).

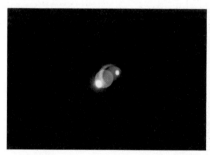

Fig. A-9. Direct illumination (conical beam).

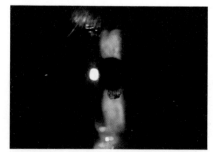

Fig. A-10. Retro-illumination: posterior corneal pigment deposits, aphakia.

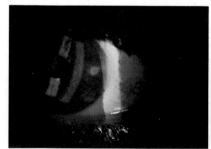

Fig. A-11. Proximal illumination (specular reflection): central corneal clouding.

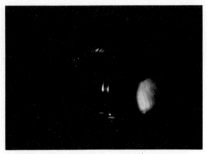

Fig. A-12. Specular reflection, high magnification.

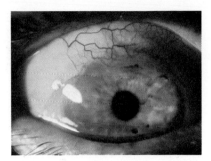

Fig. A-13. Diffuse illumination (high magnification): ruptured scleral vessel.

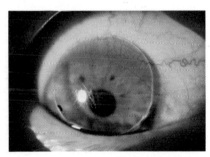

Fig. A-14. Diffuse illumination (low magnification): limbal vessel proliferation.

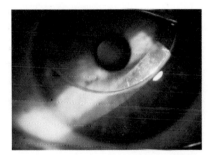

Fig. A-15. Direct illumination (medium beam): tear layer depth observable.

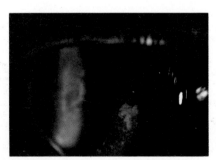

Fig. A-16. Direct illumination: mucous and debris observable.

APPENDIX B

Color plates relating to Chapter IV

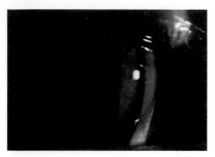

Fig. B-1. Direct illumination (medium beam): physiological edema at limbal area.

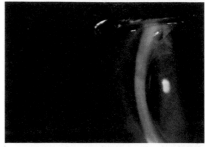

Fig. B-2. Direct illumination (medium beam): non-uniform corneal staining in peripheral areas with deeper, more serious stain a 9 o'clock.

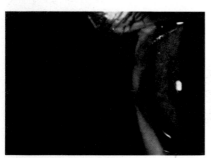

Fig. B-3. Direct illumination (medium beam): a peripherally stained corneal area at 9 o'clock, frequently also occurring at 3 o'clock.

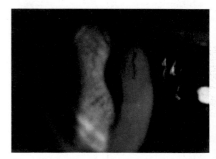

Fig. B-4. Direct illumination (medium beam): a corneal dry spot.

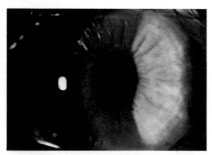

Fig. B-5. Proximal illumination (specular reflection): horizontal gray and irregualr vertical lines represent edematous areas.

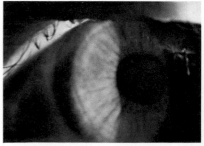

Fig. B-6. Proximal illumination: edematous areas (slight green hue).

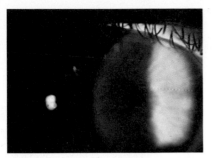 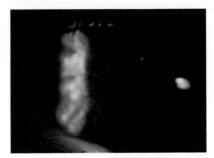

Fig. B-7,8. Proximal illumination and indirect illumination (specular reflection): the appearance of the edematous area changes when it becomes more severe. The confluence of amorphous mass formed by irregular and vertical lines.

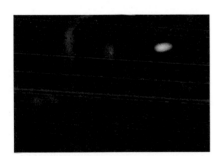 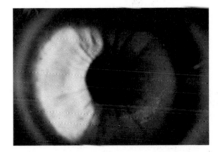

Fig. B-9,10,11. Proximal illumination (specular reflection): lens movement and improperly blended corneal stain due to excessive lens movement.

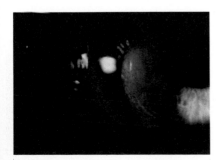 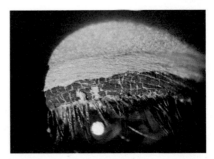

Fig. B-11.

Fig. B-12. Diffuse Illumination (high magnification): Moccara.

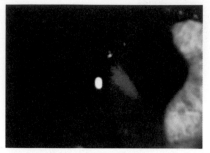 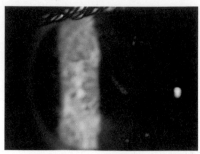

Fig. B-13,14. Direct illumination (specular reflection): superficial corneal abrasions caused by small, foreign particles or debris.

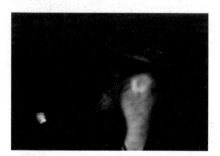 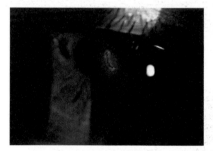

Fig. B-15,16. Proximal illumination (specular reflection): superficial corneal abrasions caused by small, foreign particles or debris.

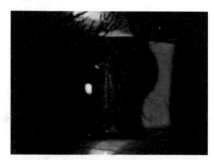 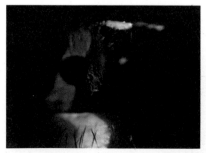

Fig. B-17,18. Direct illumination (medium beam): superficial corneal abrasions caused by small, foreign particles or debris.

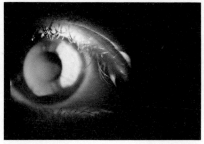

Fig. B-19. Direct Illumination, Medium Beam.

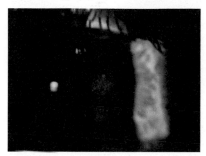

Fig. B-20. Direct illumination (medium beam): corneal abrasions induced by an apical bearing fit.

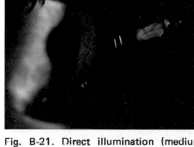

Fig. B-21. Direct illumination (medium beam): epithelial stain induced by an apical bearing fit with aperture fenestrations.

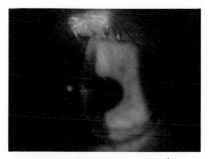

Fig. B-22. Proximal illumination (specular reflection): epithelial stain.

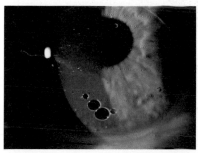

Fig. B-23. Direct illumination (broad beam): migration of bubbles beneath contact lens.

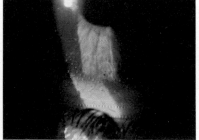

Fig. B-24. Retro and indirect illumination: small bubble formations beneath peripheral lens.

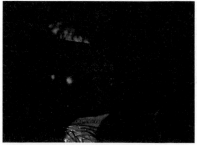

Fig. B-25. Direct illumination (medium beam): corneal scar in deratoconus.

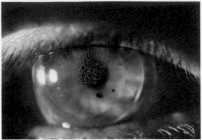

Fig. B-26. Diffuse illumination: bubbles in aphakia with post-operative iris pigment migration to posterior corneal surface.

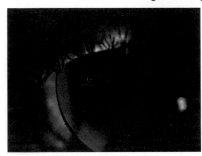

Fig. B-27. Indirect illumination (specular reflection): the epithelium indentation due to bubble retention disappears with lens removal.

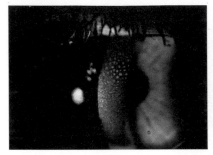

Fig. B-28. Direct illumination: (broad beam): stained areas with irregular circular design.

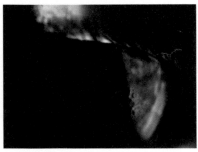

Fig. B-29. Retro illumination: epithelial dimples accentuated by corneal insult.

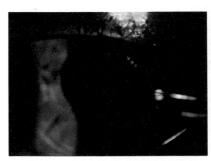

Fig. B-30. Proximal illumination: coalescence of dimpled areas resulting from irregularly shaped corneal abrasions.

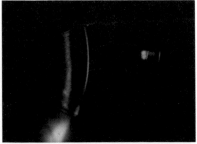

Fig. B-31. Direct -illumination (narrow beam): assessment of clearance and bearing areas.

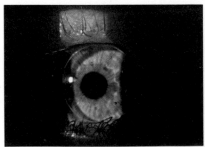

Fig. B-32. Diffuse illumination: aperture fenestrations.

CHAPTER IV

The practical
application
of biomicroscopy

The presence of a contact lens on an eye introduces a new environment under which the eye must function. Because the eye is a dynamic organ influenced by seemingly minute physical and environmental changes and conditions, a close microscopic check is necessary during *all* phases of contact lens fitting.

An external examination of the eye should be made to determine if any condition exists which would prevent the wearing of contact lenses, and an external examination cannot be considered complete without a thorough biomicroscopic examination. The biomicroscope is an indispensable instrument in the fitting of contact lenses and in the examination of the eye for the presence of minor pathological changes due to the wearing of contact lenses. It is difficult to evaluate fully the clinical effectiveness of a contact lens design when the examination is limited to the use of conventional black light and fluorescein.

The biomicroscope should not be restricted to problem cases in contact lens practice, but should be used routinely since it furnishes objective information related to the contact lens fit which is otherwise unavailable. Biomicroscopy

should be used in contact lens practice for:
1. Examination of the eye prior to the fitting of contact lenses.
2. Examination of a diagnostic control lens fit.
3. Inspection of a finished contact lens.
4. Examination of the contact lens-cornea relationship.
5. Examination of the eye after removal of a contact lens.

BIOMICROSCOPY PRIOR TO CONTACT LENS FITTING

The eyes should be examined with the biomicroscope before lenses are fitted to determine the advisability of contact lens wear.

Contact lens fitting is contraindicated when a pre-fitting biomicroscopic examination shows the presence of active corneal pathology other than keratoconus. Contact lenses are frequently the therapy of choice in this condition. Pre-fitting corneal staining with fluorescein indicates an early keratitis or ulcer. With biomicroscopy, areas of corneal dystrophy may be detected without fluorescein staining. Dry spots on the cornea are early signs of lacrimal insufficiency as in beginning kerato-conjunctivitis sicca. Lacrimal insufficiency should be suspected when fluorescein cannot be diluted by the tears.

Grosvenor (1963) considers it necessary to examine the patient for chronic conjunctivitis or blepharitis, pterygia (especially those growths which extend onto the cornea) and any other condition which might preclude the successful wearing of contact lenses (Fig. IV-1).

The presence of old corneal injuries and the characteristics of scleral and limbal vessels should be recorded as part of the pre-contact lens fitting examination since these findings are of considerable value for later comparison (Fig. IV-2).

Lester (1958) discusses a clinical procedure for the pre-contact lens fitting examination which includes a complete examination of the cornea, sclera and conjunctiva with all of the methods of biomicroscopic illumination.

While no distinction is usually made between high and low magnification for the various methods of illumination, it is assumed that each examiner will select the type of magnification which is best suited for his purposes. Low magnification should be used to establish the appropriate technique and to study a particular corneal area prior to the use of high magnification for a more detailed examination of a disturbed area (which does not require a wide field of vision nor depth of focus).

Low magnification, for most biomicroscopes, varies between 8X and 10X, while high magnification is between 16X and 20X; and these values are determined by the individual differences of the instruments. On modern biomicroscopes, the magnification may be changed quickly with a dial or a lever. Low magnification furnishes a wider field of vision and a greater depth of focus than does high magnification. The former is recommended for use with sclerotic scatter and diffuse illumination (especially when a cobalt blue filter is used to examine characteristics of the dye-stained tear layer beneath a contact lens).

54

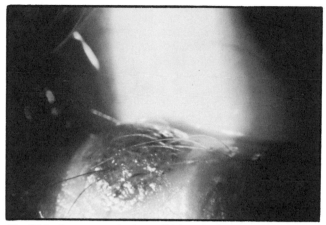

Fig. IV-1. A nevus on the lower lid found using direct illumination, broad beam, during the pre-fitting examination.

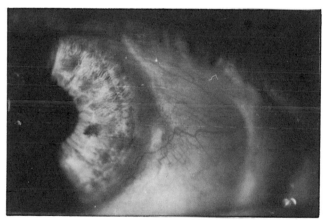

Fig. IV-2. A pterygium and vascularization found during a pre-fitting examination of the external eye.

Low magnification should be used when a large field of vision is required for a gross study: e.g., to inspect a contact lens position on the eye, as well as the dye patterns.

When low magnification is used, slight changes of patient fixation do not preclude effective examination, while with high magnification, small ocular movements by the patient may create problems. Thus, for high magnification greater than 20X, involuntary oscillations of the eyeball create interference with accurate observation.

Procedure

Use sclerotic scatter initially to examine the cornea for normal transparency.

55

Corneal scars (nebulae, masculae and perforating scars), corneal deposits and pigmented areas which are exposed by the light scattered throughout the cornea have various gray-white appearances. Corneal dystrophic areas appear as deep, irregular gray-white masses without form.

A general overall survey is made with diffuse illumination using low magnification. The angle of incident light is changed repeatedly to allow examination of the sclera and its vessels, the limbal vessels and to furnish information on corneal transparency without form or detail. The iris does appear in detail and, occasionally, one observes light reflected from the anterior surface of the crystalline lens.

Reduce the width of the beam and, with direct illumination, broad beam, examine the lid margins, eyelashes, maso-lacrimal ducts, palpebral conjunctiva and caruncle. Look for nevi, pterygia and pingueculae. Change to direct illumination, narrow beam (optical section). Traverse the cornea and examine its layers in depth.

Use retro-illumination and indirect illumination (low and high magnification) to examine for corneal scarring. Also, since contact lens wear affects the limbal vessels, a pre-fitting biomicroscopic examination should describe any unusual appearance of the limbal vessels, especially when they encroach on peripheral corneal areas.

One may frequently discover precipitates on the posterior corneal surface. These punctates may be small, circular and irregularly scattered, bilateral (although one eye may be more affected), and their color may be white or brownish-gold. They may be scattered irregularly over the posterior corneal surface or aggregated into the shape of a golden-brown vertical spindle. While pigment granules are frequently found among the aged, they are not uncommon among younger patients. One must be aware that these may be dystrophic corneal conditions (corneal guttata and Krukenberg's pigment spindle), or they may be familial traits. When found as a speckling of dust-like opacities (observed with direct illumination, medium beam, or proximal illumination) so that they present a bilateral picture of a floury cornea (cornea farinata) among the aged, they may have a relationship with glaucoma and Fuchs's dystrophy (Duke-Elder, 1965). When found among younger patients, they are usually a familial trait. I have fitted patients who have had posterior corneal precipitates (white or brownish-gold in color) with corneal lenses (although there have been no instances of corneal farinata in my practice). While these patients have had strong contact lens motivation and were able to develop wearing time, various forms of corneal interference have been found, such as early development of epithelial denudation, as well as definite prolonged pain after contact lens removal. This is similar to the subjective symptoms of "over-wearing" of contact lenses even though the wearing time had not exceeded six hours at any one time. Therefore, when any of these conditions are found during the pre-wear corneal examination, the patients should be accepted for contact lens fitting only with an understanding that their corneal state may allow only limited wear.

BIOMICROSCOPY FOR
EFFECTIVE DIAGNOSTIC CONTROL LENS FITTING

When trial lens fitting methods are used, the incidence and degree of early adaptive symptoms are not as great as they may be when a non-trial lens fitting method is used. The biomicroscope should be used to examine the trial lens fit just as one would use the instrument to examine a regular prescription contact lens fit which has been designed for the patient.

By using a biomicroscope to examine a trial lens fit, the practitioner is able to assess its characteristics so that judgment for proper selection of the lens may be made. The cobalt blue filter is used in conjunction with sclerotic scatter, diffuse illumination and proximal illumination (low magnification for all) to inspect the trial lens fit for quality of peripheral clearance, apical clearance and para-apical bearing. Direct illumination (medium beam, low and high magnification) is used to traverse the dye-stained lacrimal fluid and assess the quality of apical clearance. In contrast to conventional black light-fluorescein examination, biomicroscopy with its higher magnification and greater intensity of illumination allows immediate knowledge of the quality of the lens-cornea relationship. Biomicroscopy also furnishes information which may be used to speculate how continued wear of any particular type of clinical fit may possibly create corneal interference. Examination of the trial lens fit may also be made with white light and the types of illumination described above; however, one should not be used to the exclusion of the other.

Procedure

Use the ophthalmometer readings, external ocular and refractive findings as guides for the selection of a diagnostic control lens; place the lens on the eye and allow the tearing to subside.

Direct the patient to lower his gaze; raise the upper lid gently, and place one or two drops of sodium fluorescein from a moistened fluoristrip on the superior scleral area.

With a cobalt blue filter in place, use sclerotic scatter and diffuse illumination (low magnification) to assess lacrimal circulation beneath the lens.

Using diffuse illumination, low magnification, and direct illumination, medium beam, at an oblique angle, observe the central dye patterns and the approximate quantitative para-apical bearing.

Reduce the width of the light beam to form direct illumination, narrow beam, and focus the instrument and the incident light on the temporal lens areas. Traverse the plane of the dye stained lacrimal layer and assess the quality of the clearance and bearing areas from peripheral edge to para-apical zone, to central areas, and the para-apical and peripheral areas on the nasal side of the lens fit.

Differential Diagnosis

Air bubbles of various sizes will form under the peripheral curve areas when

57

the peripheral curve is too flat. The force of the blink will create bubbles of various sizes immediately outside the lens; some of the smaller bubbles may become retained under the peripheral lens areas, while others may migrate to the central areas. Sometimes a large bubble which may form in the inferior quadrants when the blink moves the lens down may move beneath the lens and, after a series of rapid blinks, may form several small bubbles which often migrate to the central areas and stagnate when the quality of apical clearance and para-apical bearing precludes further movement. Thus, to reduce the extent of apical clearance, use a new lens which has a base curve flatter by at least 0.50 D. (approximately 0.1 mm.), or retain the base curve value and use an optic zone diameter which is smaller by at least 0.5 mm., or any combination of these. (See also Chapter V.)

The base curve must be made flatter by at least 0.50 D., or, the optic zone diameter must be made smaller by at least 0.5 mm., or both variables must be changed in order to reduce the degree of apical clearance. (See also Chapter V.)

The base curve must be made steeper by at least 0.50 D. or the optic zone diameter must be made larger by at least 0.5 mm., or any combination of these variables may be used when one observes the absence of dye-stained lacrimal fluid in the central areas and a dark section designating apical bearing when using direct illumination, medium or narrow beam, low or high magnification, to traverse the dye-stained tear layer.

It is desirable for the practitioner to have an assortment of diagnostic control lenses properly organized according to the various fitting philosophies, as a means of conducting a thorough clinical investigation which will individualize corneal lens fitting.

A biomicroscopic evaluation of a contact lens fit should determine: (1) the width of the para-apical bearing areas, (2) the apparent circulation of lacrimal fluid beneath the contact lens, and (3) the presence of a continuous, circular dye pool around the outer periphery. Although present fitting trends reflect apical clearance philosophies which require overall lens sizes smaller than 9.0 mm., I have found patient comfort and minimum corneal interference with a lens fit which has a minimal dye-clearance pool, very narrow para-apical bearing areas, and a continuous circular dye pool on the outer periphery, along with an absence of small bubble accumulations beneath the peripheral areas, and an overall lens size which allows the lens to fit within the corneal diameter (either between the lids or slightly under the upper lid).

No matter what his fitting philosophy, by making a biomicroscopic assessment of the diagnostic control lens fit the practitioner may increase the efficiency of his contact lens service.

INSPECTION OF A FINISHED CONTACT LENS

The biomicroscope may be used to inspect a contact lens before it is worn and at any time during the fitting and post-care periods. The technique is the same in all instances and allows one to recognize lens changes induced by wearing and handling.

To inspect a contact lens when it is off the eye, attach a small piece of black velveteen material to the headrest of the instrument to form a dark background for contrast. A Q-tip, double-sided tape, or a suction cup may be used as a contact lens holder.

Use direct illumination, low and high magnification, to inspect for scratches at the junctions between all curves (there should be no radial or sponge marks created by peripheral curve forming and polishing) and to inspect the edges for uniform roundness and taper.

To inspect a contact lens for gross defects, focus the microscope in front of the piece of material suspended from the headrest (although the microscope does not have to be in focus on the material), and leave a sufficient space between the microscope and the material to allow the lens to be held, moved and turned while it is inspected so individual parts of the lens remain in focus. Use diffuse illumination and holding the lens, move or rotate it to change the angle of incident light and inspect lens surfaces. The polished surface should be smooth and consistent without cloudy or gray areas and have a high luster. A poorly polished contact lens surface has an appearance similar to that of an orange peel. Burn marks, the results of dry polishing, are slightly dense areas on the contact lens surface.

Specular reflection from the contact lens surface will reveal the normal properties of the plastic material — web-like areas will be seen which should not be mistaken for scratches. (There should be no linear or swirling scratches on the contact lens surfaces.) Cleaning or wiping scratches appear as very fine, superficial radial marks. They do not affect wearing comfort and are usually present unless the contact lens surfaces are cleaned with air drying methods.

Superficial linear scratches are often found on the contact lens surfaces and may be attributed to patient handling and contact lens storage methods.

EXAMINATION OF THE CONTACT LENS–CORNEA RELATIONSHIP

With a biomicroscope, use white light, fluorescein and white light, and fluorescein and a cobalt blue filter to augment the conventional black light and fluorescein examination techniques. The illumination and magnification of the biomicroscope makes this approach superior to the conventional black light and fluorescein technique when the fit of the contact lens is examined for corneal clearance, corneal and limbal bearing areas, and for lacrimal interchange.

Procedure

1. Use diffuse illumination, low magnification, for a gross inspection of the position and lag of the lenses and, when fluorescein is used, for a gross examination of the dye patterns. (Fig. IV-3).

2. Use direct illumination, medium or narrow beam, low and high magnification, to examine the fluorescein picture in cross-section.

3. Use all forms of illumination, low and high magnification, to inspect the cornea for pathological changes. The biomicroscope is not particularly suitable

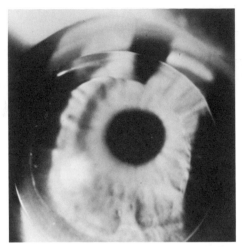

Fig. IV-3. Examination of a corneal lens fit with diffuse illumination, broad beam to inspect the relationship between the lenticular prescription element and the pupil for an aphakic patient.

for evaluating the position and lag of the contact lenses, since its greater intensity of illumination stimulates lacrimation and often causes the lens to be displaced away from what would otherwise be its regular position when it is worn.

To examine the contact lens on the eye with white light and no fluorescein:

1. Close the slit and open it slowly to form an optical section, low magnification.

2. Direct the optical section to the patient's temporal scleral area, bring it slowly toward the temporal limbus to establish sclerotic scatter, and examine the lens fit for lacrimal flow characteristics.

3. Change to diffuse illumination and examine for characteristics of the lacrimal debris and of any bubbles present beneath the contact lens, including their movement and retention (Figs. IV - 4,5)

4. Form an optical section, low and high magnification, and move slowly from the temporal toward the nasal areas of the cornea and open the slit as needed to examine clearance and bearing areas.

5. Use direct illumination, medium beam, and specular reflection, low and high magnification, to examine the front surface of the contact lens for scratches and for wetting characteristics. If the contact angle for wetting is improper, there will be immediate drying of the front surface of the contact lens in the areas where the surface is hydrophobic (Figs. IV-6,7).

6. Use direct illumination, wide beam, indirect illumination and specular reflection to examine for lacrimal debris and bubble formations beneath the

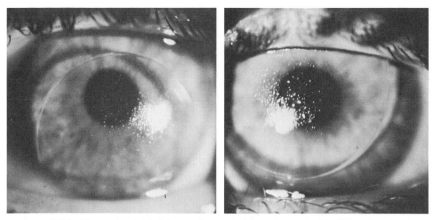

Fig. IV-4(a) (left). Lacrimal debris beneath a corneal lens observed with diffuse illumination.
Fig. IV-4(b) (right). Lacrimal debris beneath a corneal lens observed with specular reflection.

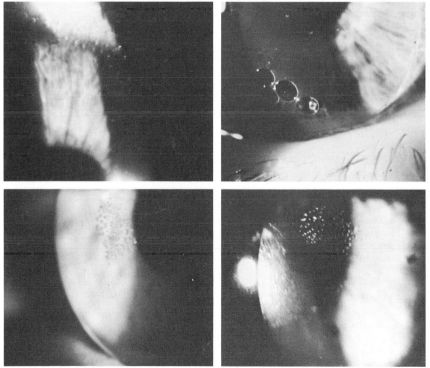

Fig. IV-5. Various forms of bubble formations.
Fig. IV-5(a) (upper left). Beneath the peripheral curve, direct illumination, broad beam.
Fig. IV-5(b) (upper right). In the outer peripheral areas, specular illumination.
Fig. IV-5(c) (lower left). In the para-apical zone, retro-illumination.
Fig. IV-5(d) (lower right). Under the apical area, specular proximal, indirect-retro-illumination.

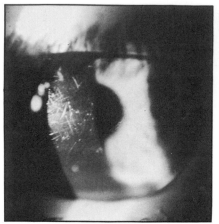 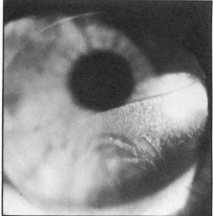

Fig. IV-6 (left). Scratches on the front surface of a corneal lens, specular reflection.
Fig. IV-7 (right). Poor wetting of the front surface of a corneal lens, specular reflection.

lens; change from low to high magnification as required.

7. Focus the microscope on the cornea and, with direct illumination, traverse the cornea and examine the corneal epithelium.

To examine a contact lens fit with fluorescein:

1. Replace the white light with a cobalt blue filter.

2. With diffuse illumination, low magnification, and a freely opened slit, form a fluorescent glow (similar to that formed using a conventional black light lamp and fluorescein). Examine for clearance and bearing areas, bubbles or lacrimal debris, and determine if lacrimal interchange is restricted in the intermediate corneal areas (particularly when an apical clearance fit is prescribed), or the central corneal areas when it is a "flat fit." With diffuse illumination, corneal intermediate zone bearing is exposed, and the approximate width of the bearing area may be estimated so that the optic zone diameter may be reduced. Similarly, one should observe the lens position as well as the characteristics of the apical fit so that he may modify the overall lens size and change the lens base curve. In time, judicious use of the instrument and experience will overcome interference created by tearing induced by the biomicroscope.

3. Use direct illumination, narrow beam (optical section), low and high magnification, and focus the microscope on the fluorescein-stained lacrimal layer. Slowly traverse the cornea from the temporal toward the nasal areas to examine for clearance and bearing areas and epithelial disturbances.

The procedures described above may also be followed when one is using white light and fluorescein. Direct illumination, narrow beam, forms an optical section through the contact lens and the cornea, and the following may be examined in cross-section:

1. A small section of the front surface of the contact lens.
2. The contact lens thickness.
3. The fluorescein-stained lacrimal line.
4. The gray line of Bowman's layer.
5. The corneal stroma.
6. The gray line of Descemet's membrane.

The fluorescein-stained lacrimal line is the brightest of all structures. Clearance areas (especially the outer peripheral corneal areas beneath the lens) have a greater column of fluorescein-stained tears — the volume decreases in the bearing areas. The fluorescein pattern observed with this technique has been compared to a wedge of fluid which increases and decreases in volume.

Fluorescein-stained lacrimal fluids beneath the central lens portions are indicative of apical clearance, and the quality of central clearance is changed by volume when the base curve of the contact lens and its optic zone diameter are altered. An alignment central dye pattern is simply minimal apical clearance. In some cases, apical clearance lens designs with small areas of intermediate zone bearing may be clinically acceptable when they do not create corneal interference.

Lacrimal tears and small bubble formations should move freely beneath a contact lens. Cluster areas of epithelial indentations are induced when small, stagnant bubble formations are retained and coalesce. Air bubbles may enter beneath a lens when there is excessive peripheral clearance, usually at the posterior quadrants. A large bubble will be flushed beneath a lens by the blink and break into smaller bubbles which, at first are connected, but then dissociate. While some bubbles are dissipated beneath the lens by further blinking and slight lens movement, others may scatter to various apical areas where they remain to stagnate, indent the epithelium, and induce corneal interference. Apical clearance, apical bearing, para-apical bearing, limbal impingement and scleral encroachment (or any combination of these) are clinical conditions which cause bubble retention beneath a corneal lens.

While subjective symptoms of pain or discomfort may be absent when the lenses are worn and the superficial epithelial layers are affected, the patient may report subjective symptoms of clouding or hazy vision; and after the lenses are removed, it may be difficult to correct the patient's vision to pre-contact lens wearing levels with any form of conventional spectacle prescription. Apparently no visual acuity loss occurs while the lenses are worn because the lacrimal layer fills the areas where there are epithelial separations and an intact refracting surface is furnished by the contact lens. Therefore, the patient may report visual disturbances after removing the contact lenses.

BIOMICROSCOPIC EXAMINATION AFTER LENS REMOVAL

One of the most important applications of biomicroscopy in contact lens fitting is that of checking for minor pathological changes of the cornea or adjacent structures which may result from wearing the lenses. A biomicroscopic examination is recommended after the contact lenses are removed since some of the more subtle conditions can be observed more easily without the lenses.

Patients will probably experience various adaptive symptoms during the first days of contact lens wear. If the adaptive symptoms persist beyond their expected duration, they are considered to be abnormal and corrective procedures must be undertaken. Faulty lens construction and fitting errors require immediate lens modification. However, some types of abnormal symptoms may not occur until months or even years after contact lenses are fitted.

Because the defensive mechanism of the eye does not warn of the impending danger, and ocular changes may occur without any symptoms (Mandell, 1965), a routine examination is necessary for all contact lens patients, whether or not subjective discomfort is present, and lens modifications should be made when ocular changes are found.

Doggart (1949) compared the cornea to a shield or an optical instrument which serves as a window through which rays pass to the media of the eye. He stated that corneal epithelial lesions may be important without necessarily constituting a threat to the efficiency of the cornea. This could characterize the corneal epithelial disturbances found among contact lens wearers.

Corneal epithelial disturbances may be induced by misdirected eyelashes, the presence of dust particles or any type of foreign body beneath a contact lens, minor traumatic corneal injuries and pathogenic organisms, including viruses, directly implanted, or derived from adjacent tissues. Disturbances of the corneal epithelium will create symptoms of pain, photophobia, excessive lacrimation and impairment of vision.

A thorough biomicroscopic corneal examination should be made when contact lenses are removed. It is necessary to use several types of illumination since each type changes the angles of incident and reflected light and exposes the cornea in different perspectives. Indirect and direct forms of illumination, low magnification, are used for a general survey; a direct form of illumination is used for a detailed study which is designed to identify and locate corneal disturbances, and indirect forms of illumination are used to examine the areas which surround and are adjacent to the disturbance.

Procedure

The types of illumination described below constitute a suggested procedure and are not listed in the order of their importance:

Sclerotic scatter, an indirect form of illumination, is used for a general survey, without form or detail, to establish the presence of corneal epithelial insult.

Diffuse illumination, a direct form of illumination, is used for a general survey, has good exposure for form and definition, and, particularly when sodium fluorescein stains the lacrimal layer, exposes the location of corneal damage.

Direct illumination uses both the broad and narrow beams to identify a corneal lesion and to determine its depth of penetration.

Indirect illumination and retro (trans) illumination are indirect forms of illumination. They are used to examine the areas which surround and are adjacent to areas of corneal insult to observe definition, translucency, consistency and pigmentation.

Corneal changes induce non-inflammatory superficial corneal epithelial changes, secondary bulbar and palpebral conjunctival injection. The limbal capillaries may become engorged and, in some instances, form peri-corneal vascularization when (1) the lens edges are improperly tapered, designed and poorly polished, (2) the lens position creates a constant pressure on limbal areas, and (3) the contact lens is allowed to encroach on the sclera (usually above the superior limbus).

Dixon (1964) described the corneal epithelium as soft, pliable, and easily molded mechanically. The absence of keratinization makes the surface easily indented. A large area of corneal epithelium is covered by the contact lens, and because of its characteristics and those of the epithelium, one may expect to observe physical and physiological changes induced by the contact lens. The severity of the changes will vary, and they are classified according to their sequential appearance.

Sodium fluorescein may be used to tint the precorneal film layer and to expose a surface irregularity, as well as a change in epithelial denudation (Berliner, 1949). The normal epithelium does not stain, but epithelial changes may cause staining when there is an interruption in the continuity of the corneal epithelium. The degree of staining is related to the severity of the damage. Non-stained epithelial edematous areas will appear grayish-white when indirect illumination and retro-illumination are used.

At onset, corneal epithelial lesions appear as small areas of edema and may progress to include areas of epithelial denudation. Almost all of the corneal changes caused by contact lenses are restricted to the corneal epithelium. Damage to Bowman's layer and the stroma is rare, since the corneal involvements are usually superficial. Corneal vascularization is noticeably absent, and this indicates that the epithelial changes induced by contact lenses are non-inflammatory. Therefore, corneal changes observed among contact lens wearers may be accepted as local changes that are not due to a general organic disturbance. There is usually a staining of the surface corneal epithelium and this may result from any or several of the following factors:

(1) Design imperfections — improper contact lens design for base curve, optic zone diameter, or peripheral curve(s); poor edge design and polish; insufficient venting (for the intermediate and outer peripheral areas) which interrupts continuous lacrimal interchange and removal of metabolic wastes; imperfect lens surfaces, with scratches, surface emulsions which have hardened, or foreign material fastened to the lens surface.

(2) Patient errors — faulty insertion techniques; poor hygiene in handling and storing lenses; re-positioning the contact lens on the cornea from the sclera.

The sequential development of corneal epithelial insult caused by the

contact lens fit or patient handling is as follows:
1. Epithelial edema.
2. Punctate.
3. Stippling.
4. Corneal abrasions and staining.

EPITHELIAL EDEMA

Doggart (1948) defined epithelial edema in its most delicate form as *bedewing*. Bedewing appears as a disturbed, wavy area resembling ripples on a water surface which will disappear quickly when the cause is removed. It may be local or general, may occur without stromal involvement, is manifested by the appearance of fine droplets or dewlike changes and appears only in a single plane (Berliner, 1949). It is best observed with retro-illumination, indirect illumination and sclerotic scatter. At the limbus, in the physiologic state, the droplets are finer and separated and are not easily recognizable. The presence of bedewing may indicate trauma, inflammation, neuropathic disturbances, raised intra-ocular pressure and corneal dystrophy. In contact lens practice, it is found to precede the formation of corneal epithelial lesions.

When epithelial edema increases in severity, (1) the surface epithelium is no longer a barrier to water, (2) the epithelial interstices may enlarge, and (3) a corneal lesion develops.

Epithelial edema disappears quickly when the cause is removed; it becomes worse when the patient is allowed to wear an improperly designed contact lens. Irregular linear forms, with or without staining and resembling infiltrates, may be observed with retro-illumination, indirect illumination and sclerotic scatter. When indirect illumination is used and the incident light is placed between 45° and 75° (proximal illumination), the incident light is scattered and the epithelial edematous areas will have a gray, dull, relucent haze which interferes with corneal luster (Berliner, 1949).

The epithelial surface of the cornea becomes edematous and cloudy within a few hours when poorly ventilated contact lenses are worn. The readiness with which the epithelium becomes edematous may be explained by its anatomy and physiology. Any condition which prevents normal physiological passage of fluids or gases through the epithelium causes stasis and resultant epithelial edema (Berliner, 1949). While epithelial edema tends to be minimal, it may lead to unusual cases wherein delayed healing leads to the development of bullous keratopathy (Duke-Elder, 1965).

Epithelial edema induced during early contact lens wearing may be a "normal" adaptive condition for most contact lens wearers because the corneal metabolism must adjust to any interference with lacrimal interchange caused by the presence of a foreign body. Boyd (1967) reported on 1,000 consecutive new contact lens patients who achieved all day wear within two days. In these patients it was possible to control the lens design variables so that all traces of epithelial edema were absent during this period; the failure rate was 3.1% (Fig. IV-12).

However, the corneal metabolism must adjust to the contact lens, and there must be a gradual development of wearing time. While it is possible for a contact lens to be worn for eight hours or longer initially, it is not a judicious procedure because subjective symptoms of pain and discomfort may be induced by the inability of the corneal metabolism to adjust quickly. I have found that the patient may become an all-day wearer when the following schedule is used: (1) Four hours continuous wear the first day. (2) Wearing time increased by one-half hour daily thereafter. Thus, the patient will develop 7½ hours of continuous wear after one week, and all-day wear will develop within two weeks. Changes in the wearing schedule may be modified according to clinical observation.

Epithelial edema may vary from very slight during the early adaptive periods, to various degrees of severity when an improperly designed lens is worn for long periods. Intercellular fluid accumulations appear as small, localized areas and become larger, circumscribed areas (usually over the apical zone) when they are allowed to develop; when there are intracellular disturbances, small vacuoles are observed.

Because of the nature of the lens-cornea relationship, edema may result. A corneal lens which is secure in position and which is not appreciably displaced by the blink may have a high degree of apical clearance and intermediate or para-apical zone bearing. Conversely, a lens which is moved excessively by the blink may have apical bearing and intermediate or para-apical zone clearance. Thus, a "tight" fit may induce physiological corneal changes when it interferes with lacrimal circulation, while a "loose" fit may induce mechanical or traumatic epithelial edema.

When a secure lens fit interferes with corneal physiology, epithelial edema is induced and intercellular staining may develop; the sequential development of superficial epithelial interference is first a punctate, followed by stippling and finally by epithelial denudation. These changes may be observed after lens removal with sclerotic scatter, retro-illumination, indirect illumination and obliquely angled indirect illumination (proximal illumination); low and high magnification may be used. Sampson (1967) stated that gross, circumscribed, edematous areas in the apical zone may be observed when the pupil is dilated using sclerotic scatter, low or high magnification, although circumscribed corneal edematous areas in the apical zone may be observed with proximal illumination when the pupil is not dilated.

Using retro-illumination and indirect illumination, low and high magnification, one may sometimes find an intracellular accumulation of fluid or small vacuoles individually scattered in the deeper epithelial layers. Because one may find it difficult to distinguish a vacuole in the deeper epithelial layers from a small bubble or lacrimal debris which might be present in the lacrimal fluid, proper diagnosis may be made when, after the patient is instructed to blink, there is no movement or displacement of the formation.

Excessively flat peripheral clearance allows air bubbles to form at the peripheral lens edges and when they migrate beneath the lens to the para-apical and apical areas, they are broken up into smaller bubbles, remain trapped beneath the lens, indent the epithelial surface and cause epithelial dimpling and edema and intercellular staining. Stagnated small bubbles may be found with a secure, apical clearance fit as well as with a loose, apical bearing fit.

The patient may experience subjective symptoms of pain, discomfort and reduced visual acuity as well as visual distress, such as clouding and haziness of vision, when the deeper epithelial layers are affected. While the edema will lessen and gradually disappear after contact lens wear is discontinued, one should remember that the eye is exposed to infection when it is edematous, and consideration for treatment should be assessed accordingly. After the edema has disappeared, lens modifications may be made and the fitting resumed.

Keratometric changes represent corneal deformation and, if the corneal bending is non-uniform in quality, it must be assumed that corneal edema is present. While Girard (1964) has suggested that a steeper keratometric finding for the flatter corneal meridian represents a quantitative edematous change, it may be incorrect to make this assumption without supporting clinical data which would describe and correlate changes of the apparent corneal thickness and posterior corneal curvatures. While a keratometric change may or may not, in itself, signify that edema is present, the presence of edema indicates that something may be wrong with the fitting situation and may result in keratometric, refractive and biomicroscopic changes. Biomicroscopy is considered the best objective procedure to determine the presence of corneal edema.

In epithelial denudation, fluorescein will stain the intercellular spaces in various hues of green in the areas which surround and are adjacent to a corneal lesion. The superficial layers will have a faint, light stain, and the deeper layers a more intense or brighter stain.

PUNCTATE AND STIPPLING

A "punctate" is a small, pinpoint, single lesion of the corneal epithelium, usually superficial, which may create pain when it affects the deeper epithelial layers (Figs. IV-8,9). It may often be accompanied by conjunctivitis, photophobia, excessive lacrimation, mild ciliary injection, and edema in the surrounding areas. It occurs when a contact lens interferes with lacrimal interchange, even before subjective symptoms appear. If the condition is not corrected, punctates increase in size and number and coalesce into large areas of staining. A series of multiple, pin-point, superficial epithelial punctates is often termed "stippling." It should be noted that punctates and stippling do not indent the epithelial surface.

A punctate epithelial lesion appears as a grayish-white area with circumscribed edema. Varying degrees of dye retention characterize the surrounding area immediately after two or more hours of contact lens wear. The lesion may not create visual disturbances; and, in cases of keratoconus, it is usually found where a contact lens has been resting constantly against the cone

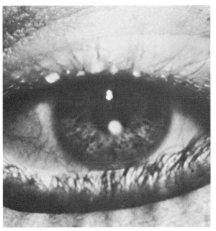 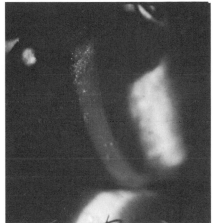

Fig. IV-8 (left). Punctate Stain (Keratoconus).
Fig. IV-9 (right). Stippling.

apex.

Sclerotic scatter, diffuse illumination and direct illumination, medium beam, are used to expose and locate the punctate. An optical section formed by the narrow beam of direct illumination is used to determine the depth of epithelial penetration, while indirect illumination and retro-illumination are used to examine the adjacent corneal areas for epithelial edema.

Contact lens wear should be discontinued until epithelial regeneration has repaired the affected area. Lens modification may then be appropriate.

CORNEAL ABRASIONS AND STAINING

Corneal abrasions due to contact lens wear may be caused by mechanical trauma or by an improper lens-cornea relationship; either of these may disturb the normal structure of the corneal epithelium and induce physiological epithelial changes such as edema and desquamation or exfoliation (Figs. IV-10,11). The severity of the epithelial disturbance is directly related to wearing time and the characteristics of the cause(s). Corneal abrasions may be the result of late diagnosis of edema caused by contact lens wear.

The cornea abrades when trauma causes an interruption or removal of a part of the epithelial surface and, for contact lens practice, "corneal abrasion" literally means a rubbing off of the epithelial cells. However, the word "erosion" has been used to describe recurrent corneal abrasion. The word "staining" refers to the fact that the corneal tissue is stained by fluorescein which has been instilled into the eye (Grosvenor, 1963). Therefore, for all practical purposes, erosion, staining and denudation are all synonymous with abrasion.

An improper lens fit, either a flat fit or a steep fit, creates a faulty

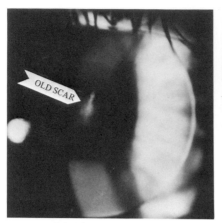 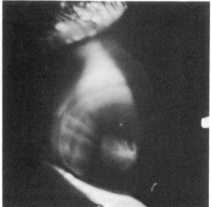

Fig. IV-10 (left). Old corneal scar.
Fig. IV-11 (right). Central corneal clouding.

lens-cornea relationship. The movement of a flat fit has a mechanical massaging effect on the epithelium which may become abrasive, and the sharp junctions between posterior surface curves (poorly blended junctions) may induce the epithelium to fold into minute branching furrows so that it wrinkles and gathers at the lens periphery. Using a biomicroscope, low or high magnification, and indirect illumination, proximal illumination or retro-illumination, one may observe irregular linear staining and/or small edematous adjacent areas. A flat fit may cause premature desquamation of the superficial epithelial cells which exposes the immature cells beneath a series of very fine, scattered, spotty lesions over any part of the cornea. Occasionally, when the inside edges of a corneal lens are improperly polished or shaped, lens movement will cause desquamation of the epithelial cells at the peripheral corneal areas, which may stain. When this condition becomes severe, it induces photophobia and lacrimation.

With a steep fit, corneal bearing areas in the para-apical zone may cause corneal deformation and/or a change in corneal structures, and the patient will experience subjective symptoms of burning, stinging, and foggy and hazy vision. Using retro-illumination, indirect illumination or proximal illumination, low or high magnification, one may observe superficial epithelial abrasions such as a punctate or multiple punctates (stippling), epithelial exfoliation or desquamation, intercellular staining intracellular vacuoles and epithelial edema. A clinical inspection and examination of a corneal lens fit and modification of the lens variables as required will prevent severe development. However, when a patient disregards instructions for the development of wearing time and overwears his lenses, severe epithelial desquamation may result. When a patient overwears a steep (or tight) corneal lens, epithelial edema is induced by the lack of corneal exposure to atmospheric oxygen, by a decrease in the hypertonicity of the tears, or by some unknown etiologic factor (Farris et al, 1967). Subjective symptoms of pain, lacrimation, photophobia and decreased vision are experienced, and the discomfort may continue twelve hours or more. Biomicroscopically, there is edema, superficial punctate(s) and staining, and the confluence of these areas often produces a large area of staining.

Corneal abrasions may reoccur (recurrent abrasions) when corneal lens wear is resumed before an epithelial disturbance is completely healed. One should examine the cornea using retro-illumination, low or high magnification, for small vesicles (intracellular vacuoles) to be certain that the healing is complete.

Aperture fenestrations are sometimes placed in corneal lenses fitted with apical clearance to dissipate stagnant lacrimal fluid accumulations beneath the apical area. Blinking will cause a corneal lens to rotate slowly, and peripherally placed apertures may cause mechanical trauma to the epithelial surface when the lens moves over corneal areas of little or no clearance. While poorly polished apertures may induce the corneal abrasion(s), if apertures are poorly polished, the patient's immediate response to pain will be lens removal without significant wear.

Mechanical epithelial trauma may be induced when a patient must recenter a corneal lens which has been displaced on the sclera. The irregularly shaped abraded areas induced are usually superficial and very transitory, and may be observed with diffuse illumination, direct illumination, medium beam, and indirect illumination, low and high magnification.

Occasionally, various substances can induce a corneal abrasion such as oils from the fingers, meibomian secretions or mucous particles may form, dry, and remain on contact lens surfaces and induce mechanical trauma to the epithelial surface when they preclude proper wetting or cleaning and become crusty formations which adhere to the posterior lens surface.

Corneal abrasions caused by faulty insertion techniques are crescent-shaped, while those caused by foreign particles (such as dust and mascara) trapped under a lens appear as swirling, irregular, radial lines which may retain fluorescein.

Sclerotic scatter and diffuse illumination are used for a general survey of corneal abrasions. Direct illumination, wide beam, is used to study the superficial epithelium; an optic section, formed by direct illumination, narrow beam, is used to determine its depth; and the surrounding areas are examined for epithelial edema with indirect illumination and retro-illumination. Both low and high magnification should be used for all types of illumination.

Phosphatase is found in cellular elements of the stroma of the normal cornea. After epithelial abrasion, a strong phosphatase reaction with lymphocytes occurs in the inter-lamellar spaces immediately underneath the affected area. The lymphocytes first increase in number quickly and then gradually decrease when the cornea returns to normal. There is cell migration to cover the injured area and mitosis reconstitutes the normal number of epithelial cells.

Although recovery from corneal abrasion occurs rapidly after contact lens removal, any abraded surface represents a potentially infectious site and the need for medical treatment should not be ignored. The patient should not wear his contact lenses until epithelial regeneration has repaired the affected areas.

71

In addition to the epithelial disturbances described above, other clinical conditions are found which are related to environment or improperly fitted corneal lenses and which preclude good wear:
1. Epithelial dimpling.
2. Limbal vessel proliferation.
3. Foreign bodies embedded in the cornea.
4. Changes in corneal curvature and refractive status.

EPITHELIAL DIMPLING

This condition presents as a group of depressed areas, or dimples, that form in the corneal epithelium as a result of the retention of bubbles beneath the contact lenses. They appear in clusters in the superior and para-apical corneal zones, are painless, produce no inflammatory reaction, induce ophthalmometer mire distortion, and may cause the patient to experience blurred vision with any form of spectacle prescription from several hours to as much as two days after contact lenses are removed (Fig. IV-12). Fluorescein will collect in the depressed areas, but most of it can be flushed out with irrigation fluid. The condition is usually associated with a securely fitting high riding lens which causes air to stagnate under the lens and, when allowed to persist, leads to interference with corneal metabolism and to epithelial edema in the adjacent areas; or with excessively flat peripheral curves which allow air bubbles to form under the peripheral lens areas and migrate to the apical areas, where they stagnate.

Dixon and Lawaczek (1962) made an exhaustive study of epithelial dimpling and reported that (1) the dimples are transient and associated with impaired tear flow under corneal lenses and (2) the exact mechanism of the formation of the dimples is unknown, but they do not appear to be due to a broken epithelial surface.

According to Dickinson (1960), these bubbles are due to corneal asphyxiation, whereas Dixon and Lawaczek (1962) feel that the air bubbles do not cause the depressions, but fill the indented corneal areas after they are formed.

Schapero (1966) commented that Dixon and Lawaczek's opinion might be a definite possibility when the blink moves a corneal lens downward so the lens edges flare away from the cornea and allow air to enter between the lens and cornea. After the blink, and when the lens returns to its original upward position, air is sealed in the superior corneal quadrants beneath the lens.

According to Schapero (1966), bubble formations seen in steep fits do not appear to be caused in the same manner, since the intermediate (para-apical) ring of touch which surrounds the central stagnant pool would tend to prevent air bubbles from passing into this area. Schapero accepted Dickinson's opinion that the bubbles are collections of gaseous metabolic waste products.

Whether or not bubble formations found beneath a corneal lens are air

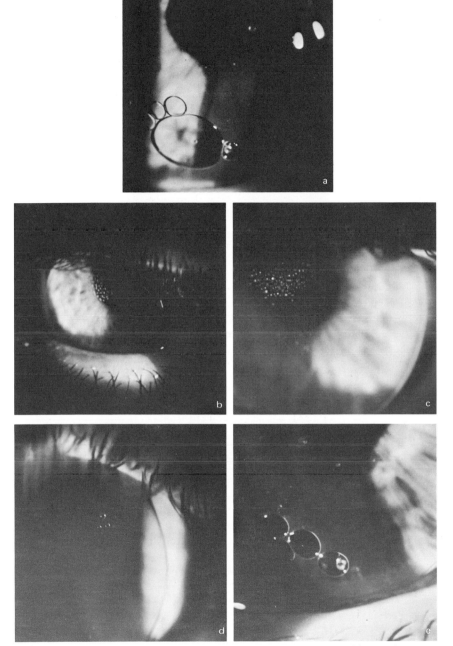

Fig. IV-12. Various types of bubble formations found beneath a corneal lens which will cause epithelial dimpling when the bubbles become trapped.

bubbles or gaseous bubbles, it is my opinion that blinking creates a constant force against stagnant, trapped bubbles so that the epithelium is indented, the interstices enlarge, and small irregularly shaped corneal abrasions of various sizes are formed which have adjacent edematous areas. The severity of the epithelial indentations as well as their differences in shape and size may be related to the bubble sizes and the force against them; all of these factors seem to be influenced by the length of time that the condition existed before observation.

When an improper contact lens design induces epithelial edema, the separation of the intercellular spaces becomes greater as the wearing time increases; and, when bubbles are retained beneath a corneal lens, they migrate toward the intercellular spaces and fill them. Thus, concave epithelial indentations are formed by a constant pressure against the bubbles by the lens. When the lens is removed, the corneal epithelial indentations are not filled with bubbles and disappear after a few hours. If allowed to remain, the areas may coalesce, cause epithelial erosion, create deeper, more diffuse epithelial abrasions, and produce pain and discomfort.

With low or high magnification, use sclerotic scatter, diffuse illumination and direct illumination, medium beam, to expose the dimpling and (when the dye is retained) use direct illumination, narrow beam, to determine the depth of epithelial penetration.

Indirect illumination and retro-illumination are used to examine the adjacent areas for epithelial edema; the corneal areas between the indentations are usually clear and epithelial dimpling often casts shadows against the iris.

Contact lens wear should be discontinued until the epithelium regenerates and the lens design is modified, if this is appropriate. Such modification facilitates improvement in lacrimal interchange and will be discussed in Chapter V.

LIMBAL VESSEL PROLIFERATION

A contact lens which impinges on the superior limbus will disrupt normal tear flow and interfere with conjunctival circulation. The tiny limbal vessels will become engorged and proliferate to the peripheral corneal areas. After contact lens wear is discontinued or the lens dimensions are modified to eliminate the cause, the vessels will recede to normal.

Irritation due to poor construction, insufficient polish of corneal lens edges, and excessive lens movement cause new vessels to form at the limbal areas. New vascularization is superficial, bright red, and is usually restricted to the area of irritation, e.g., a pterygium. Bulbar conjunctival injection may also be present.

When contact lenses induce corneal peripheral vascularization, their wear should be discontinued and the design modified. In some instances the patient may have to be refitted. Limbal vessel proliferation is not as prevalent when a contact lens is fitted which (1) is contained within the corneal diameter, (2) has minimum movement, and (3) does not create interference with corneal metabolism and transparency.

To use biomicroscopy to observe peripheral corneal edematous areas when there is limbal vessel proliferation on the cornea: (1) have the patient fixate temporally (or nasally); and (2) use indirect illumination and retro (trans) illumination, low or high magnification, to study the wavy, distorted corneal areas in the vicinity of the limbal vessels.

Dixon (1964) found that aperture fenestrated corneal lenses did not affect the incidence of limbal vessel vascularization. This finding suggests that other design components could be at fault. It is difficult to determine exactly how contact lenses causes peripheral corneal vascularization in all instances.

Corneal vascularization may be associated with the application of a contact lens to a corneal graft. However, since keratitis and iritis are usually induced in the host cornea by surgery, the vessels in the peripheral areas of the host cornea may fill and will not affect the graft after it is healed.

While the proliferation of limbal vessels on the cornea caused by an improperly fitted contact lens may lead in exceptional cases to irreversible corneal effects, I believe that the conscientious contact lens practitioner will not lose control of his fitting nor allow an improperly designed lens to be worn long enough for neovascularization to result.

FOREIGN BODY LESION

This condition may result from a chemically active or chemically inert foreign body which has invaded the cornea. It is more common among certain occupational environments, may occur at any time, and is not due to the fit of the lens or its design. The foreign body does not always cause pain (the patient is not always aware of its presence), does not create visual disturbances, and may lodge in the superficial or middle epithelial layers.

A contact lens may protect the cornea from foreign body wounds such as welding sparks, grit and debris found in certain occupations. However, small, gritty particles (mascara, dust, etc.) can be carried beneath the lens by the tears and may become embedded in the cornea while contact lenses are worn. These non-perforating injuries usually affect the epithelial layers exclusively, rarely penetrating Bowman's layer.

When fluorescein is used, one may notice an irregular film line in the area of injury, and the dye will penetrate the epithelium according to the extent of the corneal invasion. There is edema in the surrounding areas of the wound and its edges are relucent. After the foreign body is removed, epithelial regeneration is rapid.

In penetrating wounds, all the corneal layers are traversed by the foreign body, while, in non-perforating wounds, the opening does not extend toward the anterior chamber and there are no healing problems, such as corneal scarring. These may be found when Bowman's layer is penetrated.

Dixon (1964) stated that faint scratches in the epithelial surface made by foreign bodies which float into the eye and beneath corneal lenses are very common and may be considered as a normal situation.

A black light-fluorescein examination prior to biomicroscopy will expose a bright, deep, intense fluorescence where the foreign body is embedded in the epithelium. There is lighter, less intense fluorescein staining in the surrounding edematous areas. Minute foreign bodies are difficult to observe when they are colorless (such as glass). However, foreign body invasion of the epithelium usually stains with fluorescein and is properly diagnosed with biomicroscopy using sclerotic scatter and diffuse illumination technique. Direct illumination, narrow beam, is used to determine the depth of penetration. Retro (trans) illumination and indirect illumination are used to examine the surrounding areas for epithelial edema. Specular reflection is used to examine the affected area for physical characteristics of the material. Contact lens wear should be discontinued until the foreign body is removed and healing has occurred.

CHANGES IN CORNEAL CURVATURE AND REFRACTIVE STATUS

The cornea may be considered as a dynamic variable which reacts to physical pressures. Therefore, one should not be surprised when changes in corneal curvature and refractive status are found immediately after contact lenses are removed; the quantitative changes are related to time.

After the patient becomes a contact lens wearer, it is a good procedure to record corneal curvatures for each principal meridian and to refract the eye using static retinoscopy and a subjective examination during every patient visit. These values should be recorded as a permanent part of the patient's fitting history, and reference should be made to these changes as long as the patient remains a contact lens wearer.

An ophthalmometer is designed to measure curvatures from a convex corneal surface; the biomicroscope is used for an objective examination of the cornea for physiological or anatomical changes. The functions of these instruments should not be confused. It is possible that the emphasis which has been placed on ophthalmometer changes may be related to an assumption among contact lens practitioners that the contact lens fit is a good one when the flatter corneal meridian curvature changes are within plus or minus 0.50 D. of the pre-wear values.

It has been reported that steeper corneal curvature measurements found among the contact lens wearers are indicative of corneal edema (Girard, 1964) and that the steeper keratometric finding is a measurement of that edema. Yet, for these conclusions, there was an absence of supporting biomicroscopic information regarding changes in the apparent corneal thickness and posterior corneal surface. A steeper corneal curvature change may not be a measurement of corneal edema, although corneal edema may be associated with corneal curvature changes.

A contact lens may induce mechanical effects to the cornea, such as friction and swelling in the areas which are affected by lens movement; and when there is a non-uniform corneal bending (corneal warping) and corneal thickness changes, there is corneal edema. Thus, central keratometric changes make it appear as if only the central corneal areas are bending and the posterior contact lens surface is creating a forming effect on the corneal front surface. An increase in corneal thickness would be a major factor or a secondary result of the bending.

The above comments once again emphasize the need for measuring the apparent corneal thickness prior to fitting contact lenses as well as during all follow-up and after-care visits. After this information has been assembled for a representative number of contact lens wearers, perhaps it will be possible to correlate corneal curvature and refractive changes with corneal metabolic changes so that etiologic factors may be identified.

Frequently, the spectacle prescription worn by the patient prior to being fitted with contact lenses was inadequate and, although a new, pre-wear spectacle prescription was determined, it was never fitted. Therefore, it is important that at all clinical visits the patient's vision be measured with his original, as well as the immediate pre-wear, spectacle prescription, after contact lenses are removed, and the findings should be recorded. Additionally, the patient should be refracted using static retinoscopy and subjective, or manifest, examination techniques to determine the immediate spectacle prescription and visual acuity.

The results of static retinoscopy immediately after contact lens removal are unpredictable, inconsistent, and usually different from the pre-contact lens wear findings. In some instances retinoscopy may reveal dark, irregular, arcuate areas, often contained within what appears to be an impression of the contact lens on the cornea, and which resembles the retinoscopic scissors motion usually found in corneal dystrophy and keratoconus. Yet, the ophthalmometer mires may be clear; there may be no significant corneal curvature changes; the patient may report no symptoms of discomfort, and a biomicroscopic examination may show an absence of corneal interference.

A standard subjective examination is made, monocularly and binocularly, to learn if the patient's vision can be corrected to pre-wear levels. The new spectacle prescription is compared with (1) the spectacle prescription worn by the patient when he first visited the office to be fitted with contact lenses, and (2) the spectacle prescription determined when he was examined for contact lenses.

It is generally assumed that the contact lens fit is good only when the patient's vision with his pre-wear conventional spectacles returns to pre-wear levels within 30 to 60 minutes after contact lens wear is discontinued. However, I have found in many cases that when the patient's pre-wear spectacles cannot correct his vision to pre-wear levels immediately after contact lens removal and a new spectacle prescription must be used, this does not negate an otherwise good fit as long as pre-wear vision levels can be obtained with some form of spectacle prescription.

Visual acuity should be corrected to pre-contact lens wearing levels with some form of conventional spectacle prescription which is determined immediately after contact lenses are removed. Although visual acuity may vary, the refractive state eventually stabilizes so that the patient is able to interchange contact lenses and conventional spectacles without a loss of visual acuity.

When vision cannot be corrected to pre-wear levels with some form of spectacle prescription immediately after contact lenses are removed, one should be suspicious of major corneal interference. The patient should be instructed to discontinue contact lens wear for a period of three weeks, and he may be refitted with contact lenses at the end of this period according to the new keratometric and refractive values.

CHAPTER V

Biomicroscopy used to determine contact lens modification procedures

An important advantage in using biomicroscopy in contact lens practice is that diagnostic information is obtained which can be used as a guideline for contact lens modification. Biomicroscopy may be used to assess a lens fit at any time, but it is impractical to modify a contact lens fit when less than four hours of wearing time has been established, unless the fit is obviously improper.

When intermediate zone bearing, peripheral bearing, and limbal impingement interfere with gaseous and lacrimal interchange, edematous areas of the central corneal epithelium and punctate lesions are formed. Similarly, corneal insult occurs when apical bearing interferes with lacrimal interchange in the central corneal area and restricts the removal of metabolic wastes.

A contact lens may be classified by its type or by the fitting philosophy (Mandell, 1965). Lens type is determined by the size of the lens and the number of ocular curves — there are monocurve, bicurve, and multicurve lenses. The various lens types are made from a basic monocurve lens when the dimensions are changed, and these changes are related to the corneal topography and the

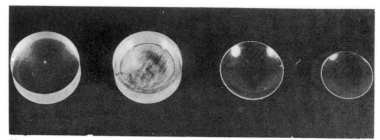

Fig. V-1. Steps in the manufacture of a corneal lens. (A) Plastic button, (B) Semi-finished blank (C) Uncut lens, (D) Finished lens.

fitting philosophy that is followed.

One should not consider himself as fitting either "large" or "small" lenses; instead, he should use clinical investigation to determine the overall lens size which is best suited for the patient. Presently, one cannot designate a corneal lens as "large" or "small", all distinctions have relative significance. While some prefer to classify a lens as "large" when its overall size is greater than 9.0 mm., and as "small" when its overall size is less than 9.0 mm., those who use the L + 2 method (for which overall lens sizes are less than 8.0 mm.) may judge corneal lenses with overall sizes as greater than 8.0 mm. as "large". Perhaps it would be more meaningful if overall lens sizes were related to how a corneal lens is fitted for its relationship to the corneal diameter and the palpebral fissure: e.g., a corneal lens may be fitted within the corneal diameter (intra-corneal diameter fit), and this may be either a between-the-lid fit (inter-palpebral fissure fit) or an under-the-lid fit.

When overall size is the basis for selecting design variables (without regard to clinical consideration of the patient's immediate needs), fitting problems may result which preclude comfort and clinical success (Fig. V-1).

CONTACT LENS FITTING PHILOSOPHIES

Contact lens fitting embraces several fitting philosophies and, while some are used to the near exclusion of others, one achieves consistent successful fitting by selecting the fitting philosophy that is best suited for each patient.

The fitting philosophies are based on a consideration of the various bearing and dimensional relationships: Apical bearing, apical alignment, and apical clearance. However, these classifications are effective, only when they are related to a monocurve lens. In recent years, advances in the design and fitting of corneal lenses have resulted in wider use of the apical clearance fitting philosophy (Fig. V-2).

Apical Bearing

If the central ocular surface lens radius (base curve) is longer than the flatter primary corneal radius, the lens is considered to be fitting flatter than the cornea ("flatter than k").

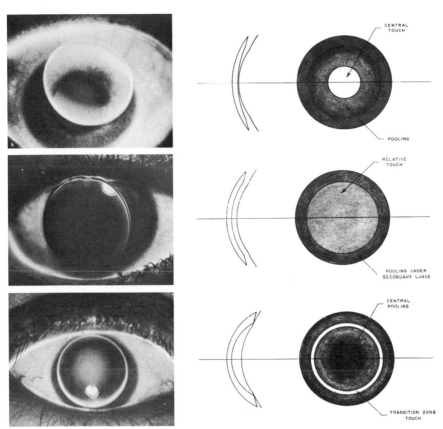

Fig. V-2. Fitting philosophies
Figs. V-2(a) and (b) (top). Apical bearing (photograph in 2(a) courtesy Solex Laboratories, Inc.).
Figs. V-2(c) and (d) (middle). Apical alignment.
Figs. V-2(e) and (f) (bottom). Apical clearance.

Historically, Touhy originally used the monocurve lens design (patented in 1950) to fit corneal contact lenses. This design was later modified by Neill, Sohnges, and Dickinson (1954). Touhy had made the contact lens base curve flatter than the flattest primary corneal meridian by 1.50 D. or more so that the curve formed is considered obsolete, although a modified version is used to fit corneal lenses in cases of keratoconus.

The original clinical use of the philosophy relied upon an appreciably flat, single ocular surface curve for peripheral corneal clearance. With apical bearing, the lens rests on the central cornea, has peripheral corneal clearance, and is rocked back and forth during blinking. According to Mandell (1965), the cornea has limited tolerance to the constant apical bearing. Since the lens movement often abrades the central cornea, wearing becomes uncomfortable and the lens is

81

ultimately rejected by the patient.

Apical Alignment

If the central ocular lens radius is made equal to the flatter primary corneal radius, the lens is considered to be fitted parallel, or on alignment with the cornea ("on K").

For this philosophy, the contact lens base curve is designed to form a plane or parallel lacrimal layer. This contact lens fit follows corneal contours as closely as possible by using two basic curves, carefully blended, with the optic zone diameter approximating the regular central corneal zone (Mandell, 1965).

This fitting philosophy has been the most popular and, until recently, the most widely used. Basically, it is a minimal clearance bicurve fit which employs optic zone diameters between 6.5 mm. and 8.0 mm., an overall lens size from 8.0 mm. to 10.5 mm., a peripheral curve usually 0.6 mm. to 1.5 mm. wide (with a radius from 0.5 mm. to 2.0 mm. longer than the base curve radius), and additional peripheral curves when there is more than usual peripheral corneal flattening or when the lens is relatively large. With the head and eyes in the primary position, the superior portion of the lens usually rests under the upper lid while the lower edge is between the lower portion of the pupil and the lower lid margin.

Although the lens is usually fitted "on K", the lens may be fitted "steeper than K" when the corneal astigmatism is 1.00 D. or greater, and "flatter than K" when the cornea is perfectly spherical.

Apical Clearance

If the central ocular surface lens radius is shorter than the flatter primary corneal radius, the lens is considered to be fitted steeper than the cornea ("steeper than K").

The lens type is usually a bicurve, although it is often made a tricurve or multicurve type when it is necessary to have improved peripheral corneal clearance.

When related to the flattest primary corneal meridian, the lens base curve is steeper by 0.50 D. or more. The optic zone diameter is from 1.0 mm. to 1.5 mm. smaller than the overall lens size. The lens size varies from 8.9 mm. to 7.2 mm. − the overall lens size variation being determined by several factors, such as pupil size, corneal diameter and topography, the amount of corneal astigmatism, the interpalpebral fissure diameter, and the lens base curve-cornea relationship. The peripheral curve radius is longer than the base curve radius, the amount being a variable. The lens position on the cornea is almost always between the lids (inter-palpebral fissure fit) and the lens positions low on the cornea, with minimum movement.

Some of the laboratory trade names for lenses designed according to this philosophy are Mini-Thin, Minalens, Sphercon, and Bayshore B-T. While they have certain differences, basically all of these lenses are apical clearance fits. Perhaps the exception is the last-named, a small tricurve lens fitted in such a way that it is supported on the cornea primarily by a wide secondary curve (Bayshore, 1962).

Whereas fitting philosophies and procedures may vary, the clinical success of any technique is directly dependent upon the maintenance of corneal transparency during and immediately after contact lens wear.

DESIGN CRITERIA FOR CORNEAL CONTACT LENSES

Black (1960) described the corneal contact lens as being a prosthesis and therefore considered the lens as capable of creating changes in the corneal anatomy similar to those created by prostheses employed elsewhere.

It should also be noted that circular shaped contact lenses do not always remain fixed in position nor move constantly in linear fashion. Nor do they necessarily rotate or float entirely on the tears.

Brucker and Carter (1961) described optimum contact lens design as ensuring (1) adequate flow of pre-corneal fluid underneath the lens and (2) absence both of excessive pressure and of excessive lens movement.

Brungardt (1962) stated that a good contact lens fit is that which provides visual acuity equal to or greater than that obtained with spectacle correction, as well as visual comfort; it must permit normal corneal and palpebral metabolism. In order to satisfy these criteria, the lens must center well, its edges must not stand off from the cornea, and the cornea must have adequate tear flow and sufficient exposure to the atmosphere.

Grosvenor (1966) listed the following criteria for contact lens design:

1. The base curve should be essentially parallel to the central portion of the cornea, thus preventing the lens form exerting pressure on the sensitive corneal apex. Also, the lens design should cause little effect on the tarsal conjunctiva.

2. The peripheral portion of the ocular lens surface should be flattened sufficiently to allow adequate exchange of tears and gases beneath the lens. It should fit loosely enough so that blinking will move it up and thus farther aid this exchange.

3. The optical zone of the lens should be large enough to keep it well centered in front of the patient's pupil, but not too large to keep it from lagging during a blink.

Grosvenor (1963a) stated that "normal physiological functions including sensitivity, transparency, water transfer and transfer of oxygen and carbon dioxide must be taken into consideration in the designing of a contact lens. Even though such optical and physical factors as visual acuity and comfort, corneal topography and adequate centration are of great importance, the final test of a contact lens depends upon the extent to which it is compatible with corneal physiology."

A contact lens must satisfy the functional needs of the patient. These needs are *critically significant*. To meet them, the lens must ensure the following: (1) maintenance of uninterrupted lacrimal interchange (venting); (2) absence of limbal impingement and scleral encroachment for any quadrant; (3) apical

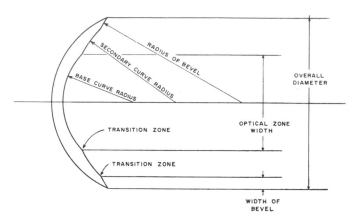

Fig. V-3. Diagram of contact lens variables (from Grosvenor).

clearance, whether it is minimum or pronounced alignment.

The *clinical* needs are *relatively significant.* The following are essential to their satisfaction:

1. The anatomic features and the metabolism of the cornea and adnexa must not be disturbed.

2. The patient must be not only comfortable, but also visually efficient when wearing his contact lenses.

3. Visual acuity must be restored to normal limits with conventional spectacles after lens removal.

4. The surface of the lens and its edges must be scratch-free and highly polished so that movement caused by lid pressures will not disturb the integrity of the epithelial surface nor irritate the perilimbal capillaries.

5. The optical element of the corneal lens should be oriented over the pupil, without peripheral curve encroachment, so that the patient will not experience monocular diplopia, flaring, and ghost images.

6. The lens should not move beneath the lower lid.

7. There should be minimum vertical displacement and change of position during blinking.

CONTACT LENS DESIGN VARIABLES

The effectiveness of a contact lens fit is determined by the individual dimensions of each design component as well as the inter-relationship between the various design components or variables. The lens must be designed so that it may be worn comfortably and with visual efficiency, will orient over the pupil, and will not interfere with corneal metabolism or corneal transparency.

The components of the contact lens design are as follows (Fig. V-3):

1. Base curve and optic zone diameter.
2. Intermediate and peripheral curve radii and their widths.
3. Lens diameter.

4. Lens center thickness.
5. Edge contour and thickness.
6. Power.

Two clinical procedures are generally used to determine the initial variables of the contact lens design, namely, non-trial lens fitting and trial lens fitting. When the former procedure is used, the ophthalmometer measurements and the spectacle prescription are sent to a laboratory by the practitioner. He may include measurement of the corneal diameter, pupil diameter, vertical palpebral fissure dimensions, and the position of the lower lid as it is related to the inferior limbus. The laboratory will design a contact lens from this information and send it to the practitioner, who must then assess its clinical effectiveness by evaluating the patient's response as he adapts to the lens. While this method furnishes a corneal lens design which will correct visual acuity and maintain a relatively good position, there is no assurance that the best lens design has been prescribed.

The alternate, more exact, and preferred method is trial lens fitting, which uses the ophthalmometer measurements and the spectacle prescription as reference points to observe the clinical performance of a series of diagnostic lenses.

Regardless of the fitting method or fitting philosophy used, it is imperative to understand how to modify contact lens design variables. When corneal insult occurs because of incorrect design, in making the appropriate modifications the practitioner may be guided by biomicroscopic findings and his knowledge of the functions of lens design components. The necessary corrective procedure may be merely a simple modification, or may involve an entirely new lens design.

If the same lens is used, the modification may consist of one or more of the following: reduction in lens size; reduction in the optic zone diameter, which is the equivalent of widening the peripheral curve(s); or flattening of the peripheral curve(s).

A new lens is required for the following modifications: change in base curve; change in power more than plus or minus 0.50 D.; increase in overall lens diameter; increase in optic zone diameter; increase in curvature of the peripheral curve(s) to a steeper, or shorter, radius; change in center thickness.

Base Curve and Optic Zone Diameter

The *base curve* is critical since it is related to prescription needs and apical clearance. Daily and Daily (1961) considered the term, *diameter,* when applied to contact lenses, to be synonymous with width, either of a curve or of the greatest distance across the lens. It is not twice the radius of curvature. The *optic zone diameter,* then, is the chord diameter of the base curve. It is the physical difference between the overall lens diameter (lens size) and the width of the peripheral curve(s), and it forms the major portion of the overall lens diameter (Baldwin and Shick, 1962). It is almost always made larger than the central corneal zone (optic cap) and the pupil (Bier, 1957). Thus, it is a critical variable for apical clearance when it is altered, and the base curve either is retained or is changed.

TABLE V–1
LENS FIT AFTER MODIFICATION OF DESIGN COMPONENTS

Base Curve	Optic Zone	Apical Clearance	Lens Fit
Steeper	Constant	Increased	Tighter
Steeper	Larger	Increased	Tighter
Steeper	Smaller	Not changed or slightly reduced	No change
Flatter	Constant	Reduced	Looser
Flatter	Larger	Not changed or slightly increased	No change
Flatter	Smaller	Reduced	Looser

Table I shows the effect on the tightness of the lens fit produced by changes in design components.

Intermediate And Peripheral Curves
The peripheral curve is a non-optical curve which has a longer radius than the base curve and is fabricated on the ocular surface so that it replaces the base curve in the peripheral areas. The radius of the peripheral curve allows the lens to stand farther away from the cornea at its edge and thus furnish an adequate reservoir of tears. The peripheral curve is made flatter than the base curve (0.5 mm. minimum difference) so that it extends from the lens periphery toward the center to form the optic zone diameter, and its width is one-half the difference between the overall lens size and the optic zone diameter.

Lens types may be defined as follows: a *bi-curve* lens has one peripheral curve and a base curve; a *tri-curve* lens has two peripheral curves and a base curve; a *quadri-curve* lens has three peripheral curves and a base curve; and a *penta-curve* lens has four peripheral curves and a base curve.

While lens types are easily distinguished by the above classification, there is no standardization of the nomenclature for peripheral curves: Manufacturers and contact lens practitioners use different terms in identification and classification. For example, the non-optical curve in the peripheral areas of a bi-curve lens may be known as a *bevel* curve or as a *secondary* curve. Similarly, when more than one non-optical peripheral curve is used, the curves may be classified according to their position on the ocular surface.

For a contact lens ocular surface, a flatter radius always replaces a steeper radius. Thus, for a base curve of 7.80 mm. (43.25 D.), a peripheral curve of 9.30 mm. (1.5 mm. or approximately 7.50 D. flatter than the base curve) will replace the base curve until the manufacturing process ends; a distinctive junction between the curves allows easy measurement of the curve widths. When a third curve is used, for example, 8.50 mm. (0.7 mm. flatter than the base curve), it will replace more of the area on the ocular surface occupied by the base curve and obscure the junction formerly present between the base curve (7.80 mm.) and the 9.30 mm. peripheral curve, but will not form an appreciably visible junction between its width and the 9.30 mm. curve because the physical difference is slight. Thus, when the junctions between peripheral curves are obscured, the lens is a *blended* lens; the blending is classified according to the quality (e.g., light, medium or heavy). While this is not particularly a good classification, it has become an established frame of reference among practitioners and manufacturers.

While some use the above procedure to fabricate peripheral curves on an ocular surface of a contact lens, others may use a different technique. For a base curve of a 7.80 mm. radius, peripheral curves of 8.50 mm. and 9.30 mm. may be required. When the 8.50 mm. curve is fabricated first, and the 9.30 mm. curve is fabricated afterwards, there will be visible junctions between all ocular surface curves. When additional curves having intermediate radii are used to obscure the junctions formed between curves, what classification should be given to the curves and the lens type? It is obvious that this is a problem for those experienced in working with standards for design, and beyond the scope of this text.

Mandell (1965) stated that the arbitrary selection of the number of peripheral curves is related to the lens design (bicurve, tricurve, et cetera) and the overall lens size. According to Grosvenor (1963), the term secondary curve refers to a curve which is just peripheral to the optical zone of a contact lens and is usually made 0.6 to 1.2 mm. longer than the base curve. The *most peripheral* curve is classified as the bevel, or peripheral curve; it is much narrower and flatter than the secondary curve, and has a radius of 11.5 or 12.5 mm.

It is my opinion that the peripheral (or secondary) curve radius and number must be based on fitting needs. A peripheral curve made 1.5 mm. flatter than the base curve has been found best for standardization for almost all of the various fitting philosophies. Occasionally, a peripheral curve made 1.0 mm. flatter than the base curve has been used to reduce lens movement and to make the lens fit more secure. It has not been necessary to use a peripheral curve made more than 1.5 mm. flatter than the base curve to make the lens fit less secure; instead, when it has been necessary to improve venting to reduce apical clearance or to loosen the lens fit, the optic zone diameter has been made smaller (or the peripheral curve width wider) by using a peripheral curve radius made 1.5 mm. flatter than the base curve.

Peripheral curve widths are decreased when their radii are more than 1.5 mm. (approximately 7.50 D.) longer than the base curve, and their widths are increased when their radii are less than 1.5 mm. flatter than the base curve to allow the lens to stand closer to the cornea.

When the peripheral curve radius is a constant for all base curves, the difference is a variable. When the difference between the peripheral curve radius and the base curve is a constant, the peripheral curve radius is a variable. For example, with a standard 12.25 mm. peripheral curve used for all base curve radii, when the base curve is 7.5 mm., the difference is 4.75 mm.; and, when the base curve is 8.00 mm., the difference is 4.25 mm. Conversely, with the use of a 1.5 mm. difference between peripheral curve and base curve radii, when the base

TABLE V–2
EFFECT OF ALTERATIONS IN P.C. RADIUS AND P.C. WIDTH

P.C. Radius	P.C. Width	Lens Fit
Flatter	Constant	Looser
Flatter	Increased	Looser
Flatter	Decreased	No change
Steeper	Constant	Tighter
Steeper	Increased	No change
Constant	Increased	Looser
Constant	Decreased	Tighter

curve is 7.50 mm., the peripheral curve is 9.0 mm.; and, when the base curve is 8.00 mm., the peripheral curve is 9.5 mm.

Alterations in peripheral curve radius and width produce changes in the lens-cornea relationship, as Table V-2 shows.

Since different methods are used in manufacturing peripheral curves, there are often differences in the fit of corneal lenses made by the various laboratories — although the peripheral curve tools used may theoretically have the same radius. Therefore, one should consistently use the trial lenses made by one laboratory.

One of several methods may be used to generate and polish a peripheral curve radius. The radius may be (1) lathe-cut and polished on the basic lens blank before the uncut lens is manufactured; (2) cut on the basic lens blank before the uncut lens is manufactured, and then polished on the uncut, or unfinished, form; (3) generated on the uncut, or unfinished, lens with either diamond or carborundum covered radius tools, and then polished; (4) polished completely on the uncut, or unfinished, lens form without prior lathe cutting or grinding.

Because the center thickness of the lens blank is not appreciably reduced when a peripheral curve radius is generated and polished on the basic lens blank, the lens is not subjected to the molecular stress and strain which occur when in this particular manufacturing process the radius is generated on an uncut, or unfinished, corneal lens. Lathe cutting and pitch polishing of the peripheral curve radius may be a more exacting, more expensive, and optically superior manufacturing method, but it may also result in fitting delays because the lens must be returned to the laboratory for modifications unless the practitioner is equipped to make pitch or wax-covered laps in his office.

Peripheral curves may be polished with radius tools covered with pitch, polishing wax, or various softer materials such as adhesive tape (waterproof and non-waterproof), velveteen, felt pads, foam rubber, or silk.

When a peripheral curve tool is covered with pitch or polishing wax, the thickness of the material does not change the radius of the peripheral curve. The exact peripheral curve radius may be generated on a tool either by lathe cutting after the pitch or wax is cooled or by forming when the pitch or wax is slightly warm.

When a peripheral curve tool is covered with a material other than pitch or polishing wax, the thickness of the material used to cover the tool makes the peripheral curve radius flatter by the amount of its thickness. One should measure the thickness of the material and make the peripheral curve radius steeper in the amount of the thickness of the material so that the peripheral curve radius will have the proper clinical value after it is polished. The tool is then said to be *compensated.* Thus, for a peripheral curve radius of 9.0 mm., one would use a radius tool of 8.7 mm. when the thickness of the covering material is 0.3 mm. However, one must expect the material to become thinner with wear and, unless he changes the pad after each use of the tool, the results will not remain constant.

Lens Diameter

The lens diameter is the sum of the widths of the optic zone diameter and the peripheral curve widths. The fit of the lens is changed when its overall diameter, or lens size, is changed. Alterations in lens size may be made with or without changes in either the optic zone diameter or base curve, or with any combination of changes. Such changes affect the lens position and fit as shown in Tables V-3,4.

Because several methods are used in fitting contact lenses, I have made no attempt to quantify numerically the changes in design variables involved in the various modification procedures. Thus, the arbitrary descriptions provided are intended only to suggest the direction of change and do not represent a precise indication of the results in the individual situation.

Edge Contour And Thickness

An important aspect of fitting corneal lenses is the quantitative value of the edge thickness and contour. When the contour fitting philosophy is employed, lens edges are made between 0.18 and 0.22 mm. thick. The edges are rounded, although they are not necessarily tapered.

Corneal lenses whose overall sizes are less than 9.0 mm. and which are fitted within the corneal diameter (and sometimes between the lids) are more comfortable when their edges are tapered and thin. The contour should begin to taper at a point 0.15 mm. from the lens edge; the thickness is between 0.12 and 0.10 mm. at this point. The tapering gradually reduces the thickness to approximately 0.03 mm. at the extreme edge, which must be rounded and highly polished for comfort.

The quality of the edge finishing may be assessed by microscopic inspection, while the contour of the edge and its thickness may be measured with a shadow profile comparator that has a millimeter measuring scale.

Although I have found the edge shape described above to be the most

TABLE V-3
EFFECTS OF MODIFICATIONS OF THE LENS SIZE AND
THE OPTIC ZONE DIAMETER

Lens Size	Optic Zone	Effect
Smaller	Constant	Makes lens fit more secure. Displaces optic zone slightly higher so that its edge moves nearer to the inferior pupil margins. Reduces the amount of lens stock that encroaches on the superior sclera and impinges on the superior limbus. May reduce lens movement.
Smaller	Smaller	Makes lens fit less secure. Decreases apical clearance. Reduces para-apical bearing and obstruction to lacrimal interchange in the intermediate zones. May increase lens movement.
Smaller	Larger	Makes lens fit more secure centrally. Increases apical clearance. Improves lens centering over pupil and may eliminate lens impingement on superior limbus and lens encroachment on superior sclera. Prevents peripheral areas of lens from encroaching on pupil areas. (Removes flaring, ghost effects, and monocular diplopia.) May eliminate or reduce vertical displacement.
Larger	Constant	Makes lens fit more secure. Eliminates lagging of lens. Improves meridional orientation.
Larger	Smaller	Makes lens fit more secure, although lens position may be slightly upward. Reduces apical clearance. Reduces amount of para-apical bearing. Eliminates lagging of lens.
Larger	Larger	Makes lens fit more secure. Increases apical clearance. Prevents peripheral areas from encroaching on pupil areas. (Removes flaring, ghost effects, and monocular diplopia.) Eliminates lagging of lens. Improves meridional orientation.

TABLE V-4

EFFECTS OF MODIFICATIONS OF THE
LENS SIZE AND THE BASE CURVE

Lens Size	Base Curve	Effect
Constant	Steeper	Makes lens fit more secure. Increases apical clearance. Reduces vertical displacement. Improves lens centering over pupil.
Constant	Flatter	Makes lens fit less secure centrally. Reduces apical clearance. Reduces amount of intermediate zone bearing and removes obstruction to lacrimal interchange in the para-apical corneal areas. (Improves venting.)
Larger	Constant	Makes lens fit more secure. Improves geometric centering of lens on cornea. Reduces lens movement.
Larger	Steeper	Makes lens fit more secure. Increases apical clearance. Improves lens centering over pupil. Reduces lens movement.
Larger	Flatter	Makes lens fit less secure centrally, but more secure generally. Reduces apical clearance. Improves lens centering over cornea. Reduces amount of intermediate zone bearing and removes obstruction to lacrimal interchange in the para-apical corneal areas. (Improves venting.)
Smaller	Constant	Reduces the amount of lens stock that encroaches on the superior sclera and impinges on the superior limbus. Displaces optic zone slightly higher so that its edge moves nearer to the inferior pupil margins. May reduce lens movement.
Smaller	Steeper	Makes lens fit more secure. Increases apical clearance. May increase para-apical zone bearing. Reduces the amount of lens stock that en-

(Cont.)

91

(Continued from preceding page)

		croaches on the superior sclera and impinges on the superior limbus. improves centering of lens over pupil.
Smaller	Flatter	Makes lens less secure peripherally and centrally. Reduces apical clearance and intermediate zone bearing. Improves intermediate zone venting. May cause lens to lose geometric centering on cornea.

successful in my practice, each practitioner has his own concept of what constitutes a good edge shape. What would be considered optimum by one practitioner could be totally rejected by another. This seems paradoxical when one considers how much emphasis is usually placed on obtaining a "good" edge shape. However, Mandell (1965) discovered that various edge shapes were tolerated by the test patients, but that well-tapered edges with little edge stand-off on the concave side were *preferred* by the majority of the subjects. To quantify the edge contour, he used an adjustable, L-shaped template which allowed the lens edge to fit into it and created a boxing system similar to that used with spectacle lenses. Mandell found that, for a myope wearing a standard lens design and size, the optimum edge has a contoured profile and gradual thickness reduction; the lens edge is 0.16 mm. thick at a point 0.5 mm. from the outer edge, 0.2 mm. thick at a point 0.14 mm. from the outer edge, 0.08 mm. thick at a point 0.05 mm. from the outer edge, and 0.03 mm. thick at the outer edge itself.

Two methods which employ the biomicroscope may be used to inspect lens edges, direct magnification and projection magnification.

Direct Magnification

1. Using low or high magnification, open the biomicroscope diaphragm to its maximum width.

2. Hold the lens either between the fingers or in a small-diameter suction cup (or a holder which will not obscure the lens edges).

3. Look through the microscope and move the lens nearer and farther away, up and down, until it is in focus.

4. View the lens edge that is visible and observe the contour of the edge as the lens is tilted and slowly moved nearer and farther away. Rotating the lens, repeat this procedure until the entire edge has been inspected.

5. Inspect the lens edge for lathe marks (poor polishing), scratches, indentations or elevations, and appropriate edge contour design.

Projection Magnification

1. Reduce the room illumination.

2. Using low or high magnification, open the biomicroscope diaphragm to its maximum width.

3. Hold the lens either between the fingers or in a small-diameter suction cup (or a holder which will not obscure the lens edges).

4. Move the lens nearer and farther from the microscope until a shadow of the edge is in focus on either an adjacent wall surface or a small, white paper mounted on a wall near the microscope.

5. Slowly rotate the lens and observe the edge contour.

While this second method may be successful as described, it is enhanced when used in conjunction with the projection shadow-profile magnifier.

Comment is in order for those who assess the quality of a finished corneal lens edge by (1) rotating the lens edges *around their tongues*, or (2) placing the lens on *their* eyes to determine if the edge is finished properly. The first procedure is very unsanitary and cannot provide the objective results obtained with instruments which are designed for this purpose. The results of the second procedure are influenced by individual corneal sensibilities. The technical and scientific advances in contact lens practice have made unhygienic and primitive procedures unnecessary.

Supplemental Design Components

Gordon (1961) stated that the major considerations in corneal contact lens fitting are the physical relationship of the lens to the cornea and the amount of tear interchange. Lacrimal interchange requirements may be satisfied, generally, by determining the proper relationship between lens design components and the physiological needs of the cornea. However, there are often instances when certain limiting factors (such as corneal diameter, pupil size, palpebral fissure vertical diameter, lid and corneal sensitivity, lid tension, and corneal topography) preclude using conventional fitting methods and lens designs. In such instances certain design changes may increase venting and thus aid lacrimal interchange requirements. These changes may include placing a series of holes in a lens (aperture fenestration) or creating a series of channels on the inside lens surface (chamfer venting) to eliminate stagnant lacrimal pooling and bubble formations beneath apical bearing areas.

Haynes, Brungardt, and Pollock (1960) described "venting" as the "establishment of the flow of precorneal fluid between the ocular surface of the contact lens and the cornea, so that there will be no embarrassment of the physiological functions and mechanisms of the cornea and the adjacent paralimbal and limbal regions of the eye." Modification of contact lenses to improve lacrimal interchange generally involves reduction of the overall lens size and the optic zone diameter. Sometimes when it is necessary to reduce these values further, the modification may change the lens position and create such undesirable effects as flaring, monocular diplopia, and patient discomfort. Therefore, it may be preferable to solve the fitting problem by retaining the existing lens values and introducing aperture fenestrations or chamfers. However, the center thickness of a contact lens is not affected by the placement of the apertures, while the center and the edge thickness must be increased when channels are constructed.

Aperture Fenestrations

Historically, Bier (1957) discovered that the placement of an aperture in a scleral lens was helpful in postponing or reducing Sattler's veil, a condition which had previously been responsible for limiting wearing time. Bier postulated that the following criteria for aperture placement are applicable to corneal lenses: constant flow of lacrimal fluid beneath the lens, access of atmospheric oxygen to the cornea, and provision for the escape of dissolved carbon dioxide (Fig. V-4).

Bayshore (1962) described the use of a central aperture in an apical clearance lens to ventilate the apical pool. According to Bayshore, one or several holes may be used to interrupt the continuity of a contact lens surface. Individual aperture diameters should be at least 0.20 mm. wide (although they may be made as large as 0.30 to 0.35 mm.) so they break the surface tension of the tear layer during blinking, and allow tears and metabolic debris to pass through them.

Using empirical procedures, I have developed the following use of apertures:

1. Four holes are equidistantly placed immediately inside the optic zone diameter. (The placement of one aperture at the geometric center is uncommon.) The apertures are between 0.20 and 0.35 mm. wide when the overall lens size is less than 9.0 mm., between 0.20 and 0.25 mm. wide when the overall lens size is greater than 9.0 mm., and between 0.25 and 0.30 mm. when it is greater than 10.0 mm.

2. Additional apertures are added, similarly placed, if indicated by clinical investigation.

3. Aperture fenestrations are used when a base curve change or optic zone diameter change (or both) will eliminate a fitting problem, but will also destroy the clinical effectiveness of the lens fit.

I use a miniature drill press, 250 r.p.m., with a reverse motor action to drill the apertures in a contact lens. The bit is used for only six fenestrations, and is then discarded.

The apertures should be normal to the surface in all lens areas, have a straight bore, with surfaces free of any irregularities. Biomicroscopy with high magnification will reveal any imperfections. The surfaces should be polished after the apertures are bored. It is not necessary to polish the interior walls of the apertures when they are made according to the procedures described above. An aperture fenestration will cause patient discomfort when it is insufficiently polished at its edges on the lens surfaces or when the fabrication was made other than normal to the surface. It is important for the lens position to be changed during fabrication to allow the bit to enter the lens perpendicular to the surface. Aperture fenestrations will induce discomfort, regardless of the size of the holes, when they do not conform to the conditions previously described. I disagree with the contention of Korb (1962) that apertures over 0.15 mm. induce patient

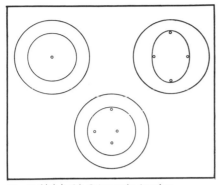
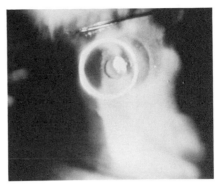

Fig. V-4(a) (left). Schematic drawing.
Fig. V-4(b) (right). Aperture fenestration in a scleral lens.

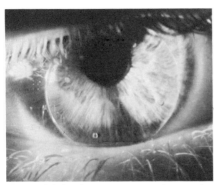
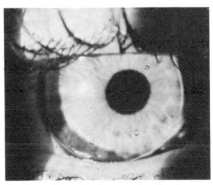

Fig. V-4(c) (left). Four aperture fenestrations placed equidistantly from each other in a corneal lens.
Fig. V-4(d) (right). Three aperture fenestrations in a corneal lens not equidistantly spaced.

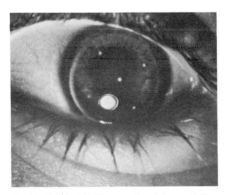
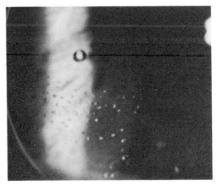

Fig. V-4(e) (left). Fluorescein picture of five aperture fenestrations in a corneal lens. (The apertures are not clogged, the dye stained tear layer is seen beneath them; spillage occurs only when the blink forces stagnant fluid through the apertures.)
Fig. V-4(f) (right). Bubble formations may remain trapped beneath the lens in certain areas until lens rotation moves the apertures over the stagnant fluid.

discomfort and create lens warpage, since apertures made smaller than 0.15 mm. have been found unsatisfactory for general use although they are sometimes employed with overall lens sizes smaller than 8.0 mm.

Occasionally, when observed with black light and fluorescein, apertures may appear to be so filled with debris that they clog and prevent lacrimal flow. However, biomicroscopy with diffuse and/or retro illumination may show that the apertures are not clogged. The fluid flow may be reduced because (1) fluid pooling is insufficient in the immediate area of the hole, or (2) the aperture is too small to break the surface tension of the fluid.

While aperture fenestration is generally introduced to augment venting, it is particularly useful when indicated in apical clearance fitting.

The use of aperture fenestrations does not preclude the development of epithelial edema, although they frequently help the patient to overcome some of the early adaptive problems. Stagnated lacrimal pools may be forced through the apertures by the hydraulic action of the blink. Thus, aperture fenestrations may be used to augment venting needs during the early, or initial, fitting periods and, in my opinion, may be retained when they do not create either visual distress or mechanical trauma to the epithelial surface.

Frequently, in my practice, when aperture fenestrations have been prescribed for corneal lenses fitted within the corneal diameter with apical clearance, their use has reduced the severity of initial adaptive symptoms, and the patient has developed as much as seven or eight hours of continuous wear without discomfort. Therefore, aperture fenestrations sometimes may be the only remedial modification available for solving a venting problem.

After the adaptive symptoms have been overcome and the patient has become an all-day wearer, the corneal lens with aperture fenestrations may be replaced with one of identical design, but without aperture fenestrations. This is usually done if visual distress results from excessive tear spillage through the apertures, or if at night the patient is aware of irregular reflections surrounding lights, et cetera, caused by light scatter off the walls of the apertures.

Apertures may induce mechanical epithelial edema when there is excessive lens movement and not enough apical clearance. When a lens moves over a corneal area of little or no clearance the break in capillarity can cause friction and trauma of the superficial epithelial surface with denudation. This condition may be characterized by linear abrasions or irregularly shaped and scattered punctates on the epithelial surface. These may stain and, when observed without the use of fluorescein, appear as greyish-white areas. It must be noted that this type of lens fit may cause mechanical trauma even without the fenestrations. With direct illumination and low or high magnification, one may use the biomicroscope to observe the degree of the denudation. When the incident light is moved nearer to the patient to form a more oblique angle ($55°$ to $75°$), the use of indirect proximal illumination will help expose adjacent edematous areas (Fig. V-5).

Chamfer Venting

By definition, "chamfer" means channel or furrow, and, when applied to

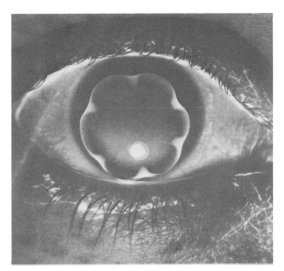

Fig. V-5. An apical clearance fit within the corneal diameter and between the lids.

contact lenses, the term describes the fabrication of grooves on the ocular surface, from the lens periphery to the central optic zone area, to create a passageway for tear flow and facilitate lacrimal interchange.

Chamfer venting has been used here and abroad for both scleral and corneal lens designs (Gordon, 1961). The Butterfield Para-Scleral Lens employed a series of grooves to form a passageway for lacrimal interchange, while the Stimson Corneal Lens had a series of protrusions extending from the inside lens surface whose purpose was to provide continuous lacrimal interchange. Vent-Air, SpiroVent, and AstroCon are corneal lens designs which utilize the chamfer principle. Chamfer venting is used more successfully with larger lenses, and a chamfer vented lens may be augmented with aperture fenestrations.

LENS FIT PROBLEMS AND THEIR CORRECTION

Whatever fitting philosophy is involved, the lens-cornea relationship will be affected if the lens fit is too secure centrally, too loose centrally, too secure peripherally, or too loose peripherally, or if it exhibits a combination of two of these clinical problems.

When a contact lens contours the cornea only in certain areas to support the lens position and pulls radially away from the corneal surfaces in other areas, the fit may be described as providing proper venting. A corneal lens fit is unsatisfactory if it exactly matches the corneal contour because it interferes with lacrimal flow, allows retention of metabolic wastes and reduces the oxygen supply to the cornea (Fig. V-6).

Because corneal topography cannot be measured exactly with current instrumentation, corneal reaction to contact lens wear is assessed after lenses are

97

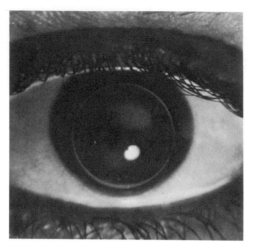

Fig. V-6. Lens fit too secure centrally.

removed by (1) keratometric examination, (2) biomicroscopic examination, and (3) refraction.

Lens Fit Too Secure Centrally

A lens fit that is too secure centrally is produced by an apical clearance lens which has one or more of the following characteristics: (1) the base curve is too steep; (2) the optic zone diameter is too large; (3) there is excessive bearing in the intermediate corneal areas; (4) the peripheral curve is too steep.

Clinical Findings

The lens appears firmly fixed in position over the pupil. Only minimum vertical displacement upward or downward occurs during blinking, and the lens usually retains its position of geometric orientation over the cornea. Characteristic findings of black light-fluorescein examination are apical pooling, bearing areas in the para-apical corneal zones, and a continuous band of fluorescein-tinted tears around the peripheral lens areas. After the lenses have been worn four hours or more, bubble retention may be observed beneath the central lens areas. When the bubbles coalesce, corneal abrasion may result. The patient usually experiences burning and stinging, and other forms of visual distress. After the lenses are removed, it is often difficult to achieve with conventional spectacles visual acuity which is equal to pre-wear levels. Interference with visual acuity experienced after contact lens removal has been called *spectacle blur*. It is a symptom of metabolic interference, may persist for several minutes or several hours, and sometimes can be eliminated with a different spectacle prescription. The effectiveness of this new prescription is very transitory and it may be unsatisfactory after a few hours. When vision cannot be corrected to pre-wear levels with any form of spectacle prescription, the patient

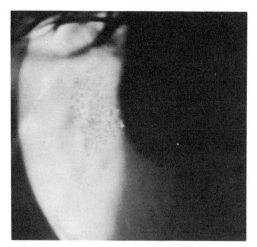

Fig. V-7. Bubble formations beneath a corneal lens fitted too securely centrally.

should be instructed to discontinue contact lens wear for an extended period, after which he may be refitted.

The factors of apical clearance and a zone of para-apical bearing may create interference with lacrimal interchange beneath the lens and induce metabolic changes. The stagnant bubble formations beneath the lens usually indent the epithelium. Biomicroscopy is used to detect apical bearing, lacrimal interchange deficiencies, and epithelial dimpling and edema (Fig. V-7).

Use sclerotic scatter and diffuse illumination to examine the bubble formations in the central areas beneath the lens for size, position, and movement, and to study their surrounding areas.

Change to direct illumination, medium beam, and while the microscope is focused on the tear layer (this is simplified when the tears are tinted with 2% sodium fluorescein), traverse the tear layer from the temporal to the nasal areas and observe clearance and bearing areas. Focus the microscope on the areas of bubble formation and alternately use indirect illumination and retro illumination to examine for epithelial edematous areas.

Remove the lens and examine with an optic section the areas of epithelial dimpling and determine their depth. Areas of epithelial edema appear as localized, small, irregularly shaped areas adjacent to the bubble formations. The edematous areas will appear grayish-white, cloudy, and slightly obscured when there is no staining.

Characteristically, the apical clearance design does not produce bubble retention, stagnant central lacrimal pooling, and epithelial dimpling. A small lens design may fit firmly in position, geometrically centered over the cornea, and its narrow width of para-apical bearing does not always interfere with lacrimal interchange. However, in some cases the lens fit may be improper and yet appear to be normal when examined with fluorescein and black light, and biomicroscopic examination may not expose edematous areas or interruption of the epithelial surfaces. Yet, after the lens is removed, dark, irregular, arcuate areas which are contained within what appears to be an impression of the contact lens on the cornea can be observed with static retinoscopy. Ophthalmometer measurements may be as much as 1.00 D. steeper for the flatter primary corneal meridian, and visual acuity equal to pre-wear levels cannot be obtained. It would be correct to assume that the lens fit is too secure and has induced corneal changes.

Modification Procedures

Apical clearance and the width of the para-apical bearing areas must be reduced to eliminate interference with lacrimal interchange. One may consider it judicious to make these changes in small amounts so the effect of each change may be observed; if further modifications are required, they may be continued until the problem is corrected. When the optic zone diameter is made smaller, apical clearance is reduced, as is the width of para-apical bearing areas.

To reduce the optic zone diameter, use the existing, or a flatter, secondary curve radius (from 0.3 to 0.5 mm. flatter) to improve venting. When one chooses to reduce the optic zone diameter so that the modification does not create a major change of the lens position, he may employ a radius of curvature which is slightly steeper than the existing peripheral curve and slightly flatter than the base curve. The peripheral curve tool used for this procedure is covered with a soft material (velveteen or silk) to *blend* the transition angles between curve junctions. This modification will reduce the optic zone diameter and automatically increase the width of the peripheral curve(s) when the lens size is retained as a constant.

The optic zone diameter may be reduced by 0.3 mm. when the lens size is less than 9.0 mm., and by 0.5 mm. when it is larger than 9.0 mm., especially if the lens design is a contour fit. It is questionable whether the fitting problem will be eliminated if the optic zone diameter is reduced in amounts less than these values.

Another method may be used to make the lens fit less securely, that is, reduction of the overall lens size from 0.2 mm. to 0.4 mm. Also, a series of flatter peripheral curves may be used to form a parabolic edge curvature which will facilitate lacrimal interchange. In the modification of the peripheral lens edges, the procedure of using a flat radius first and then progressively steeper radii will automatically reduce the transition angles between curves and obscure their definition (blending). The peripheral lens areas will then have several flat curves with small widths and minimum edge stand-off and thus aid venting.

To produce a parabolic edge contour, one may use a radius of 17.0 mm. for a width of 0.1 mm., 15.0 mm. for a width of 0.1 mm., 12.0 mm. for a width of 0.1 mm.

The successful fabrication of a parabolic edge design depends upon the presence of sufficient lens stock. A lens may have insufficient edge thickness to allow this modification to be made successfully, since the use of flatter curves at

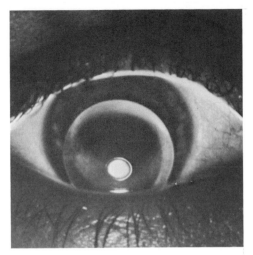

Fig. V-8. Lens fit too loose centrally.

the peripheral areas may remove plastic and reduce the overall lens size. Therefore, this type of modification may necessitate the fabrication of a new lens with a center thickness great enough to permit the overall lens size to be retained.

When it appears that a further reduction of the optic zone diameter will cause the inferior lens edge to encroach on the pupil, it is necessary to make a new lens with a base curve which is flatter by at least 0.50 D. (approximately 0.1 mm.). This will reduce apical clearance and provide a larger optic zone diameter. When the base curve is made flatter, the lens power must be compensated for in the amount and direction of the change.

Lens Fit Too Loose Centrally

A lens fit that is too loose centrally (Fig. V-8) is produced by an apical bearing lens which has one or more of the following characteristics: (1) the base curve is too flat, (2) the optic zone diameter is too small, (3) the peripheral curve or curves are too flat and/or too wide, (4) the lens size is too small, (5) the center thickness is too thick for the power.

Clinical Findings

The lens position may be positioned on or slightly below the inferior limbus. The lens edges may stand away from the peripheral corneal areas and thus produce bubble formation and stagnation beneath the central areas. When part of the lens is covered by the lower lid, there is interference with lacrimal interchange and gaseous exchange. A base curve which is too flat or an optic zone diameter which is too small, or both, may produce apical bearing. Although a lens is fitted according to the alignment philosophy, apical bearing may

101

develop when the flatter corneal curve becomes steeper in the early months of wear or when the lens base curve flattens.

Apical bearing causes a looser lens fit. Excessive lens movement induced by the blink may produce small punctate abrasions (stippling) or irregular epithelial abrasions (without form or pattern). When an epithelial area which is edematous adjoins one of stippling or abrasion, severe corneal abrasions and ulceration may result.

With black light and fluorescein, there is marked peripheral clearance and deep fluorescence; the apical areas are dark. Occasionally, irregular epithelial staining is observed. The patient may be more aware of the lens, although he may experience no pain or other distress. However, there may be photophobia, burning, and stinging. The lens may move off the cornea or out of the eye. Vision with conventional spectacles after contact lens wear is usually less than pre-wear levels.

For biomicroscopic examination, while the lens is worn, tint the tear layer with sodium fluorescein and use direct illumination, medium beam, low and high magnification, to traverse the cornea. Focus the microscope on the tinted tear layer and observe apical bearing areas, which appear as dark areas without fluorescence. Use sclerotic scatter with low magnification, and diffuse illumination, indirect illumination and retro-illumination with low and high magnification, to observe movement of lacrimal debris and the formation and retention of small bubbles in the apical areas.

After the lens is removed, use diffuse illumination, indirect illumination and retro-illumination with low and high magnification to examine the limbal vessels for engorgement and any extension of the limbal vessels to the corneal peripheral areas. Examine the peri-limbal vessels with diffuse illumination, low and high magnification. Have the patient change fixation approximately 10° to 15° temporally. Then reduce the width of the beam and change the angle of incident light to approximately 45° to 60° temporally. Use indirect illumination and retro-illumination, low and high magnification, to examine the limbal vessels in the nasal portions of the cornea. Then, reversing the procedure, examine the limbal vessels in the nasal portions of the cornea. Then, reversing the procedure, examine the limbal vessels in the temporal corneal portions.

Use diffuse illumination and indirect illumination with low and high magnification to detect areas of corneal epithelial erosion, which have any one or combination of the following characteristics: (1) a series of small punctate lesions within the apical bearing area, (2) epithelial edema in the immediately adjacent areas, which appear as grayish-white irregular lines, (3) denudation of corneal epithelium (stained areas). Wearing the lens without modification may induce further epithelial changes, such as deep abrasions, edema, and corneal ulceration (Fig. V-9).

Modification Procedures

Restore apical clearance with a *new* lens in which the base curve is 0.50 D. steeper (usually 0.1 mm.), with prescription compensation, and/or the optic

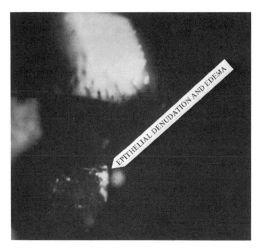

Fig V-9 Epithelial denudation and edema induced by a corneal lens fitted too loose centrally, observed with indirect illumination and specular reflection, high magnification.

zone diameter is 0.5 mm. larger for a modified contour fit or 0.3 mm. larger for a non-contour fit.

When the optic zone diameter of the new lens is larger and it has the peripheral curve width of the old lens, the lens size will automatically be increased. For example, if the old lens had a lens size of 9.5 mm. and an optic zone diameter of 7.5 mm., its peripheral curve width was 1.0 mm. When the optic zone diameter is changed to 8.0 mm., and the peripheral curve width of 1.0 mm. is retained, the lens size becomes 10.0 mm. Conversely, if the optic zone diameter is changed to 8.0 mm., and the lens size is retained (9.5 mm.), the peripheral curve width becomes 0.75 mm.

When the lens is positioned either on or below the inferior limbus, make the new lens size larger (by either 0.3 mm. or 0.5 mm.) in combination with the procedures described above. A peripheral curve which is 0.8 to 1.2 mm. longer than the base curve may be used to form the new optic zone diameter. The width of the new peripheral curve will be influenced by the remedial procedures already discussed.

When the center thickness is too great for the power, the lens is moved across the cornea by the blink. A new lens, made thinner by 0.02 mm. to 0.03 mm., may produce a more secure lens fit. The center thickness value of the thinner lens must be compatible with the overall lens size, the power, and the width and radius of the peripheral curve. Since an alteration in center thickness may also change the characteristics of the edge thickness and design, it may be advisable to use a lenticular construction when it is necessary to reduce the center thicknesses for certain powers so that the thickness and design of the edge

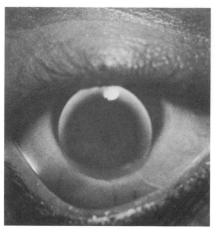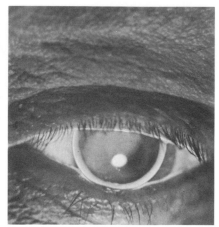

Fig. V-10 (left) and Fig. V-11 (right). Corneal lens fitted too securely peripherally.

may be retained, for example, for plus power lenses.

Lens Fit Too Secure Peripherally

A lens fit that is too secure peripherally is usually a *high-riding* lens in that part of the lens covers the cornea while another part impinges on the superior limbus or encroaches on the superior sclera. The cause is one of the following: (1) the overall lens size is too large; (2) the peripheral curve or curves are too wide and/or too flat, with the result that excessive edge standaway causes the lens to be displaced upward by the blink. When this occurs, it is likely that the optic zone diameter is too small (Figs. V-10,11).

Clinical Findings

The lens is fixed in position high on the cornea. There is insufficient peripheral clearance in those areas where the lens impinges on the superior limbus. This frequently causes the limbal vessels to fill and proliferate into the peripheral corneal areas. Occasionally, there is also conjunctival injection.

The high lens position is characteristic of an "on K" fit for corneal astigmatism of 2.00 D. or more (spherical base curve lens), especially for a lens of high minus power. Mandell (1965) stated that the cornea can easily support the lens in a high position because the center of gravity tends toward the posterior side of the lens. When the lens position is high the optic zone diameter often encroaches on the lower pupil areas and the patient may report visual distress concomitant with monocular diplopia.

With fluorescein and black light one observes deep lacrimal pooling in the superior quadrants; there is usually an absence of fluorescence in the areas of insufficient peripheral clearance. There is deep, continuous peripheral clearance beneath the inferior lens edges, especially when the lens stands away from the cornea.

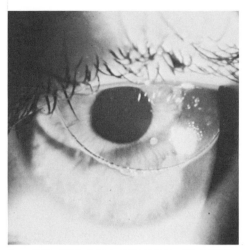

Fig. V-12. High riding corneal lens with bubble formations at the lower areas. Direct illumination broad beam, low magnification.

The patient may be aware of the lens during blinking when the lens edges are (1) thick and round, (2) square and sharp, or (3) thin and poorly polished, or when they stand away appreciably from the eye and form an oblique angle at the lens edge (ski-nose edge shape). Tear stagnation may cause photophobia, burning, and stinging.

This type of fit induces epithelial edema, stippling, dimpling, and superficial vascular changes in the superior limbal areas. Biomicroscopic examination with sclerotic scatter, low magnification, will expose stagnant bubble formations beneath the lens. Use diffuse illumination, low and high magnification, to examine the bubble formations and the lacrimal pooling in the superior corneal quadrants: (1) Examine the bubble spacing (Fig. V-12) and observe changes in the position of the bubbles when the upper lid is retracted and the patient looks downward, (2) Study the appearance of the superior limbal vessels to detect changes from the findings of the biomicroscopic examination made before fitting. After instilling fluorescein with the lens in place, use direct illumination, medium beam, low and high magnification and focus the microscope on the tear layer. Traverse the cornea and examine for apical clearance and bearing areas. Examine for limbal vessel proliferation as well as general peri-limbal vascular changes by means of indirect illumination, retro-illumination, diffuse illumination, and direct illumination, medium beam, low and high magnification.

After the lens is removed, examine the areas of epithelial dimpling with direct illumination, medium beam, and with an optic section, narrow beam, low and high magnification, determine their depth. Indirect illumination and retro-illumination, low and high magnification, are used to examine corneal edematous areas.

Modification Procedures

The modification often employed first is reduction in overall lens size, with retention of all other design components. The peripheral curve width is thus automatically reduced, and while reduction in size may correct the lens impingement on the superior sclera, it changes the lens position upward relative to the pupil. As part of the same modification, one may make the edges thinner, thus removing the tendency of the upper lid to grip the lens and move it upward. (In lenticular constructions this problem is minimal.)

Although the above modification may be successful, in making any change one must be guided by the individual clinical condition. As a general rule, a high lens position is the result of improper base curve selection and occurs when a spherical base curve is fitted "on K" to correct with-the-rule corneal astigmatism in excess of 1.50 D. The lens is in alignment with the flatter, horizontal corneal meridian, its edges stand away from the steeper vertical meridian, and the blink moves the lens upward. One can correct this fitting problem by using a steeper base curve (retaining the optic zone diameter or making it larger) and a smaller lens size; the lens will fit within the corneal diameter and, usually, within the palpebral fissure.

The base curve is made from 0.50 to 1.00 D. steeper, according to clinical findings. However, whenever possible, trial lenses should be used to determine the quantitative change. When the corneal astigmatism is greater than 2.50 D., toric base curves should be considered. Aperture fenestrations may be used to satisfy venting requirements.

To facilitate lens centering, one may find it helpful to make a new lens which has a larger optic zone diameter (between 0.3 and 0.5 mm.), since apical clearance increases when the base curve dimension is retained and the optic zone diameter is increased.

A prism ballast design with increased center thickness may be used to lower the lens position. The prism is between 1.0 and 1.5 prism diopters; the base curve is made steeper; and the optic zone diameter may be either retained or made larger, causing it to be displaced 0.5 mm. above center toward the apex of the prism to center the optical element of the lens over the cornea. An unequal peripheral curve width is thus formed.

One may also use a new lens which has a steeper base curve, larger optic zone diameter, smaller overall lens size, and thinner center thickness to center the lens over the cornea.

Lens Fit Too Loose Peripherally

A lens fit that is too loose peripherally is produced by a decentered lens which has one or more of the following characteristics: (1) the base curve is too flat; (2) the optic zone diameter is too small; (3) the lens size is too small; (4) the peripheral curve is too flat (Figs. V-13, 14, 15).

According to Grosvenor (1963a), a loose fit may result when a lens is fitted with a steep base curve which touches only at the periphery, so that the lens is moved appreciably by the blink. The displacement of lenses may be due to

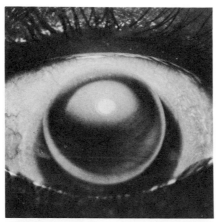

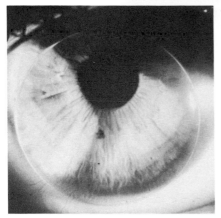
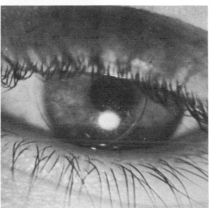

Fig. V-13 (top). Lens fitted too loose peripherally.
Fig. V-14 (left). A corneal lens fitted too loose peripherally; diffuse illumination, low magnification.
Fig. V-15 (right).Nasal displacement of corneal lens fitted too loose peripherally.

corneal asymmetry, particularly decentration of the corneal apex and non-uniform corneal flattening.

Clinical Findings

The lens does not center well. The displacement may be nasal or temporal, high or low. The peripheral areas often encroach on the pupil and induce visual disturbance. Often, the lens moves during blinking. Excessive lens movement may cause superficial epithelial disturbances such as punctates, stippling, and irregular linear staining. Occasionally, discomfort and visual distress result when mucous and lipid deposits form on the lens surfaces. Conjunctival injection may develop after relatively short periods of contact lens wear. The peri-limbal vessels may become engorged and proliferate into the peripheral corneal areas.

Lens movement may cause photophobia, lid irritation, and lid edema. The patient may report a need to "squint" to prevent the lens from moving off the cornea or out of the eye.

Biomicroscopy will reveal the epithelial disturbances resulting from this type of poor fit, and it will show lacrimal interchange to be unaffected. Bubbles which migrate beneath the lens are quickly dispersed. However, peripheral air pockets beneath the lens occasionally fill with a large bubble or several small bubbles; the latter may remain when the peripheral curve is too flat.

With the lens in place, use sclerotic scatter and diffuse illumination to examine for metabolic interference and deposits on the lens. Mucous particles may have various shapes and formations. Their movement pattern can be seen clearly after fluorescein staining. If the lens surface is coated with these particles, changes in surface wetting characteristics will be observed.

The metabolic disturbances which may occur have various characteristics: (1) Areas of epithelial denudation appear as irregular, grayish-white sections on the corneal epithelial surface. They vary in depth and are usually present where apical bearing and excessive lens movement have affected the cornea. These areas will stain with flourescein. (2) Punctates and stippling caused by lens movement, may be found over various corneal areas.

Conjunctival injection and irritation of the lid margins, resulting from lens movement and poorly designed edges, are examined with diffuse illumination (low and high magnification).

With direct illumination, narrow beam (low and high magnification), optic section is used to evaluate the relationship between the corneal periphery and the peripheral curve(s).

Grosvenor (1963a) described the technique for observing this relationship in cross section with an optic section after fluorescein staining. He stated that the tear layer beneath the peripheral curve appeared wedge-shaped (like a prism), and evaluated the peripheral curve according to its biomicroscopic appearance:

1. In a proper relationship, the base of the wedge is toward the periphery.

2. The peripheral curve is too steep (insufficient venting) when the base of the wedge is toward the center rather than toward the periphery.

3. The peripheral curve is too flat (edge standoff) when the base of the wedge is toward the periphery and is very wide.

After the lens is removed, with direct illumination, narrow beam, low and high magnification, examine all abraded corneal areas to determine the depth of the abrasion. Indirect illumination and retro-illumination, low and high magnification, are used to examine epithelial edematous areas, which appear grayish-white when they are a part of the erosion complex and stain with sodium fluorescein, and changes in the peri-limbal vessels.

Modification Procedures

A new lens is usually required to provide centration over the pupil and cornea. It must have a larger overall size and/or larger optic zone diameter with or without steeper base curves, a minimum center thickness, and thin, tapered edges.

The modification of lens dimensions may consist of one or more of the following changes: (1) overall lens size larger by 0.3 to 0.5 mm., (2) base curve steeper by 0.50 D. or more and with prescription compensation, (3) optic zone diameter larger by 0.3 or 0.5 mm., (4) values of the peripheral curve and its width adjusted as indicated by biomicroscopic evaluation.

One will find that the use of trial lenses will facilitate determination of the necessary changes.

CHAPTER VI

Biomicroscopy photography

Biomicroscopy photography can make valuable contributions to contact lens practice. The illustrations which it provides may be used (1) to study contact lens designs and evaluate their clinical effectiveness so that modification procedures may be determined; (2) to create a pictorial case history; (3) to document corneal pathologic conditions, supplying a pictorial record which may become valuable evidence for medicolegal use; and (4) to enhance or replace classroom or lecture materials.

One of the first to employ photography successfully in conjunction with biomicroscopy was Goldman (cited by Duke-Elder, 1962), who attached a photographic apparatus to the slit lamp and was thereby able to calculate the volume of the anterior chamber. Mazow (1961) used a photo attachment with a Thorpe biomicroscope to photograph the external eye; a system of absolute stereophotography of the slit lamp optic section was developed by Norton (1964). Bronson (1966) described a technique for photographing the external eye through a single lens reflex camera mounted to one of the eyepieces of a biomicroscope; he used a silicon-controlled rectifier to increase the illumination of the slit-lamp bulb for adequate illumination for color photography. Niesel (1966), using the Scheimpflug principle and a Philips electronic flash, adequately photograhed the anterior segment of the external eye with the Haag-Streit, 900 slit lamp. Employing a method previously described by Schirmer (1965), Cohen (1966) placed a microscope slide obliquely in the path of the slit lamp beam, splitting the beam into two parts by refraction, so that the external eye could be photographed after the microscope was displaced to the side.

In 1961, Gambs developed an effective method of biomicroscopic photography. For this method, the binocular microscope of the Gambs Model 750 instrument is removed and replaced by a photo-attachment secured in position on the arm which is used to support the microscope (Goldberg, 1964). A Zeiss extension tube (63 mm., 1:45) is secured to a mount fitted with a screw extension so that it may be fastened into the position normally occupied by the microscope on its supporting structure. This extension tube is fastened into a single lens reflex camera box and thus replaces the camera lens system. A 20-inch cable release attached to the camera is held in one hand and the other hand is used to adjust the slit-lamp and the camera position. The observer sights monocularly through the camera. Standard methods are used to establish the type of biomicroscopic illumination required to expose the condition to be photographed.

The high illumination of the slit lamp furnishes sufficient lighting for the use of color film (Kodak High Speed Ektachrome Artificial Light – Type B – EHB 135, ASA-125). A shutter speed of 1/60th second is used; the magnification of the resultant picture is 1.25X.

With the photo-attachment secured in position, the following procedure is used:

1. The camera and the lamp housing are aligned according to the usual biomicroscopic technique.
2. The patient is instructed to direct his gaze to a pre-determined fixation point; the fixation light of the instrument may be used.
3. The lamp housing is moved to the required angle, the slit opening is adjusted, and the entire instrument is moved with the joy stick to establish the type of illumination required.
4. When the particular corneal area to be photographed is in focus, the shutter is triggered by pressing on the cable release.

One may create variations in the general lighting effect of the areas observed by changing the diaphragm opening of the Zeiss extension tube. For this method, best results are obtained when the tube is opened to its maximum setting (1.0), while the slit-lamp diaphragm is adjusted appropriately.

For the above method I have substituted one that allows the photograph to be taken with no interruption of the examination or modification of the regular biomicroscopic technique. For this method I have employed a Gambs Model 1000 photo slit lamp which has the following design characteristics: A Leica camera box, without the lens system, is attached to the microscope immediately

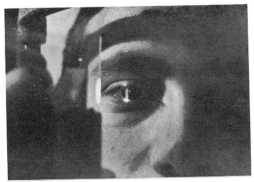

Fig. VI-1. A microscope slide is held obliquely in the path of the slit-lamp beam and serves to split the beam into two parts by refraction.

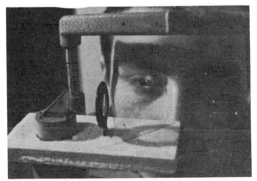

Fig. VI-2. Balsa wood carrier in place on the illuminating arm of the Bausch & Lomb slit lamp.

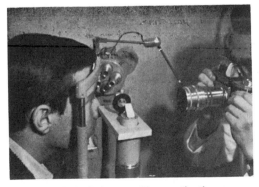

Fig. VI-3. Method photographing a patient's eye.

Photographic methods described by Cohen (from Optometric Weekly).

above the eyepiece (a bayonet type is used for proper orientation). The observer sights through the microscope binocularly in much the same way he would when using general examination procedures.

When ready to photograph, one interposes a reflex-mirror in the optical path of the left microscope by lowering the handle adjacent to it. Now the right eye views through the right microscope and the left eye observes the focusing and framing to determine the proper conditons for photography. The illumination should be turned to the brightest position. (A foot pedal is depressed to increase the illumination.) The shutter is then triggered by pressing on the cable release which is attached to the camera box.

Since the observer views through the binocular microscope of the instrument, he can take a picture quickly and easily at any time during the examination. This system is a *permanent* photographic arrangement, since the lens system is fitted permanently within the structure of the microscope. The concentrated light from the slit-lamp covers a circular field the size of the iris diameter. Although photography of the anterior part of the external eye has been accomplished with this method, Gambs has used it with a Hruby lens and gonioscopic contact lenses to photograph the fundus and the anterior chamber.

All of the methods described above limit the reflection of the lighting and thus do not interfere with patient's comfort.

While these methods are excellent for photographing the anterior segment of the external eye, the illumination is insufficient to photograph an optic section. However, one may make photographs while using the biomicroscope with low and high magnification; the diaphragm of the instrument, constructionally modified, furnishes a field depth on the film which corresponds to that obtained in the microscope with the standard eyepieces (magnifications of 10X and 20X) and 4 D. of accommodation amplitude (Gambs Company).

The characteristics of the binocular viewing and photographic system with the Gambs Model 1000 Photo Slit-Lamp are listed in Table VI-1.

TABLE VI–1
MEASUREMENT DATA FOR BINOCULAR METHOD

	Magnification	
	Low (1X)	*High (2X)*
Linear magnfication	*1.5X*	*3.0X*
Corresponding visual magnification (proximate)	*10.0X*	*20.0X*
Photographed-field width	*16.0 mm.*	*8.0 mm.*

I have found that best results are obtained with a shutter speed of 1/15th second and Kodak Ektachrome High Speed Film (ASA-125), Artificial Light, Type B. Also, while this system was employed to investigate techniques for black and white photography, it was found that better black and white prints were obtained with a black and white negative made from a color transparency.

Gambs has also designed a Polaroid camera attachment to be used with the Model 1000 Photo Slit-Lamp. For this system, the lens system of the Polaroid camera is replaced with a bayonet type attachment which secures the camera to the attachment on the instrument. While this is advantageous in that it provides a means of making finished prints quickly, I have found that the illumination system of the instrument is inadequate for good color reproduction; and, while black and white prints may be made with this system, using a shutter speed of 1/15th second, the details are not as well-defined as they are in photographs obtained with the Gambs photographic system previously described.

The Haag-Streit biomicroscope employs a photo attachment which has the following characteristics:

1. Viewing is binocular through the microscope; the picture is visualized through the camera, which is a single lens reflex camera body attached to the biomicroscope.
2. The camera mount attaches to the microscope and has a photograhic objective, adapter ring, camera holder, camera body, and interchangeable photograhic objective — 1:1 and 1:2. With 1X magnification the optical image measures 24 by 36 mm.; with 2X magnification, 12 by 18 mm.
3. An electronic flash is used for illumination, and a special bulb (3400° Kelvin), for photography. Artificial light film (High Speed Ektachrome, EHB-135, ASA-125, Artificial Light, Type B) is best for proper color reproduction.
4. The photograph is made through the prism of the special interchangeable mirror, and the images are reversed on the film.
5. The slit-lamp must be inclined 15° so that the light falls on the lower part of a special mirror, illuminating the object uniformly.
6. A single lens reflex body with a bayonet cap for proper orientation is used, and this can photograph only the anterior segment of the external eye.

The Zeiss Company manufactures two adjuncts for biomicroscopy photography: (1) a photo attachment for its conventional biomicroscopes, and (2) a photo slit-lamp which is designed to photograph the anterior segment of the external eye as well as the details of an optic section. It should be noted that only the Zeiss photo-slit lamp is designed for the latter purpose.

Photo attachment characteristics: The camera, whose mount attaches to the microscope, has a photographic objective, camera holder, adapter ring, camera body, and interchangeable photographic objectives (1:1 and 1:2, or both). The aperture of the photographic objective is situated centrally between the two observation apertures of the corneal microscope so as to provide a large depth of focus. The magnification obtained with the photo attachment may be increased to 1:4 by using a special 2X supplementary objective for the 1:2 photographic objective. The high intensity electronic flash which is used is synchronized with the camera shutter and is adjustable.

Photo slit-lamp characteristics: The new photo slit-lamp is similar to the

115

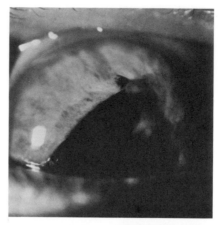

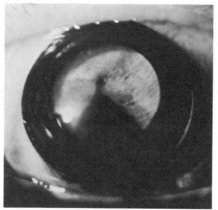 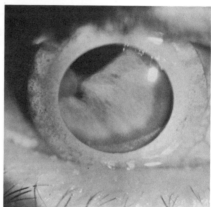

Fig. VI-4 (top). Sphincterotomy and scar tissue.
Fig. VI-5 (left). Opaque periphery corneal lens fitted for initial clinical investigation.
Fig. VI-6 (right). Early stages of fitting a cosmetic corneal lens.
Photographic history of cosmetic corneal lens fitting for sphincterotomy.

other instruments manufactured by the Zeiss Company. There is an anterior segment illuminator which is a pilot light used to locate the position of the light reflex and the electronic flash on the cornea so that the reflex will not appear in the picture or obscure the condition to be photographed; this illuminator is regulated for brightness by a recoss disc with different apertures at the light exit. The flash generator and transformer is a highly developed electronic apparatus which supplies energy for the bulb and flash tube in the slit illuminator, the bulb and flash tube in the anterior segment illuminator, and the bulb in the fixation device. Stereo pictures may be taken when the small beam splitter is interposed between the body of the microscope and the binocular tube. However, this technique is not recommended because it produces a 50% loss of light, and the

TABLE VI–2
EXPOSURE CHART*

Type of photograph	Illumination aperture	Anterior segment illuminator	Photo objective	
			Aperture	magnification
Survey photograph with ground-glass screen	9		45	1X 2X
Survey photograph with wide slit	3-9		64	1X 2X
Photograph with narrow slit (0.1 mm.) of weak opacities (normal lens)	5	2	11	1X
of medium opacities	3	2	11	1X
of strong opacities (and cornea)	5	4	22	1X 2X
Photograph in retrograde light (slit 0.1 mm.)	9	2	11	1X

* Courtesy Carl Zeiss Co.

maximum opening is smaller than that in the objectives in standard use. Successful photography requires the achievement of the proper relationship of photo aperture and illumination aperture widths. Recommendations for setting the proper apertures on the recoss disc are listed in Table VI-2.

The following are the criteria for successful biomicroscopy photography: (1) faithful color reproduction, (2) correct exposure, and (3) clear identification of the subject photographed.

The recent developments by Gambs, Zeiss, and Haag-Streit have simplified and enhanced biomicroscopy photography. It is possible to photograph the external eye as it is observed with various types of illumination when the biomicroscopes designed by these firms are used with their various photographic arrangements.

Although employing the techniques of biomicroscopy photography may be difficult during the initial periods, skill comes with practice. Turning out an excellent picture has been for me a source of excitement and satisfaction, and I have found biomicroscopic photographs to be an effective record when reviewing certain contact lens fitting problems   the periods which have been

117

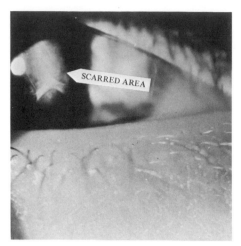

Fig. VI-7. Corneal scar in keratoconus.

given to study of the color transparencies have been rewarding ones.

With the development of the Nikon Zoom-Photo Slit Lamp Microscope, it is now possible to photograph the images projected from the microscope finder. The instrument's magnification can be readily changed from 7X to 35X by turning a dial which employs a zoom-in principle. Photograhic attachments utilized in taking slit lamp photographs include either a Nikkormat or Nikon F camera, an electronic flash tube adapter with a condensing lens, a vertical photo-tube, electronic flash tube, a power cord, and an electronic power supply.

The Photographic Assembly: The camera is mounted on the vertical photo-tube so that its prism housing faces the release side. When the examiner uses his right hand to grip the joy stick the photo tube should be mounted on the left hand bushing. This will allow the right hand to grasp the joy stick and to focus the instrument while the left hand operates the shutter release. For either camera the shutter speed should be set at 1/60 second. However, for the Nikkormat the "X" synchronization contact should be used, while for the Nikon F the "FX" setting is employed.

Because a background illumination filter has a central transparent portion and a peripheral diffusing surface, it should be substituted for the blue-green color filter. Care should be taken so that the filter's central transparent portion and the slit lamp are aligned in the same direction. When this alignment is obtained, the light passing through the filter's transparent portion is emitted as a light bundle with sufficient depth of focus for accurate viewing while the light passing through the diffusing surfaces of the upper and lower halves evenly illuminates the surrounding areas of the slit image. The illumination filter thereby furnishes a lighted background which may be used as a reference for location of the primary photographic subject. Also, the use of this filter allows a simultaneous recording of the outer orbital sections as well as the area

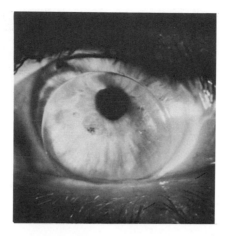

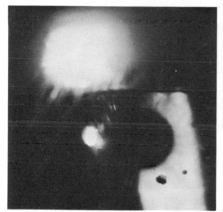 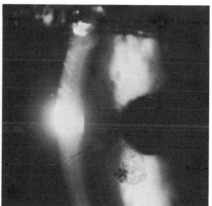

Fig. VI-8 (top). Diffuse illumination, low magnification.
Fig. VI-9 (left). Retro-illumination, low magnification.
Fig. VI-10 (right). Retro-illumination and indirect illumination, high magnification.
Posterior corneal surface pigmentation induced resulting from aphakia surgery.

illuminated by the slit section. However, the filter has no useful purpose when higher magnification photographs are made, since it degrades the picture contrast. When the Hruby lens is lowered into position the fundus may be photographed.

For white light photography, high speed Ektachrome film is used (Daylight type, ASA 125). To photograph, push the release grip down on the vertical photo-tube side. This allows the built-in mirror to move down into the microscope's optical path so that the shutter release is coordinated with the electronic flash.

The proper use of this flash is an important variable for obtaining the best

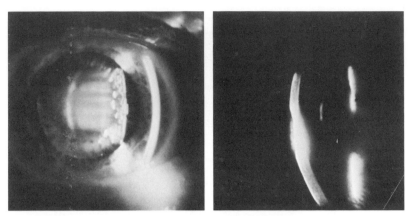

Fig. VI-11 (left). Coronary cataract; slit illumination (Photo courtesy Carl Zeiss Co.)
Fig. VI-12 (right). Keratomycosis slit illumination. (Photo courtesy Carl Zeiss Co.)

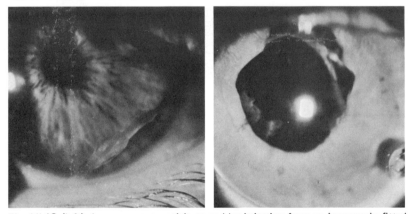

Fig. VI-13 (left). Large mucous particle caused by irritation from an improperly fitted corneal lens.
Fig. VI-14 (right). Scleral lens fitted for aphakic eye, with remnants of capsular material.

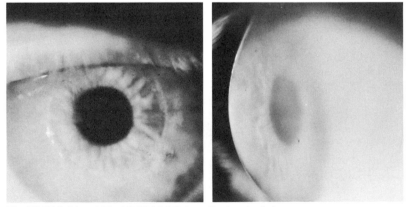

Fig. VI-15 (left) and Fig. VI-16 (right). Lamellar keratoplasty.

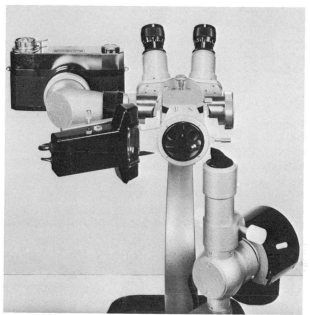

Fig. VI-17. Zeiss slit-lamp with camera attachment and electronic flash.

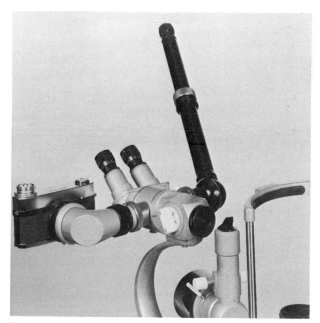

Fig. VI-18. Zeiss slit-lamp with camera attachment and observation tube.

121

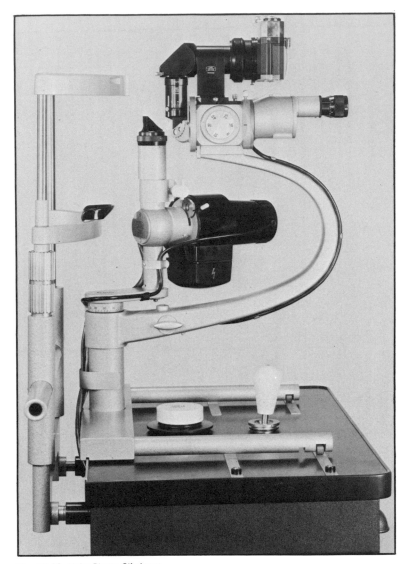

Fig. VI-19. Zeiss Photo Slit-lamp.

BIOMICROSCOPY PHOTOGRAPHY

possible pictures. It has five different positions which may be used depending upon the region to be photographed and the magnification to be used. It should be noted that it is necessary to use more light, or a greater intensity of the electronic flash, when the magnification is increased. The following table is used for quick reference to assure that the proper flash intensity is used for photographing the various parts of the eye:

Figures represent

Flash output (intensity) x Film speed (ASA)

Location	Magnification	0.7–1.0	1.1–1.6	17–2.5	2.6–3.5
Conjunctiva		35	70	140	280
Iris		50	100	200	400
Fundus		200	400	800	1600
Cornea	Wide Slit	150	300	600	1200
	Narrow Slit	200	400	800	1600
Crystal-line	Wide Slit	200	400	800	1600
lens	Narrow Slit	400	800	1600	3200

Black light photography of the eye may be accomplished with the use of cobalt blue filter. The film recommended for this purpose is Anscochrome 500, ASA 500; however, the film should be developed using procedures designed for ASA 1000 (Kaps, 1969). However, the use of this film does create a problem; it is too fast for photographing the anterior segment of the eye. Because Anscochrome 500 fails to photograph one portion of the eye, both the selection of film and the determination of whether the instrument will be used for white light or black light photography become variables of increased importance to the practitioner.

For my biomicroscope, the camera is always loaded and ready for action.

Bibliography

Adler, F. H.: Physiology of the eye. Clinical application. 3 ed. C. V. Mosby Co., St. Louis, 1959

Ashton, N.: Corneal vascularization. In the transparency of the cornea. Edited by S. Duke-Elder and E. S. Perkins. Blackwell Scientific Publications, Oxford, 1960

Baldwin, W. R., and Schick, C. R.: Corneal contact lenses. Fitting procedures. Chilton Co., Philadelphia, 1962

Baud, C. A., and Balavoine, C.: L'ultrastructure de la membrane de Descemet et de ses derives pathologiques(stries hyalines). Ophthalmologica(Basel) 126:390-4, Nov 53

Bayshore, C. A.: Report on 276 patients fitted with micro-corneal lenses. Apical clearance and central ventilation. Amer J Optom 39:522-3, Oct 62

Berens, C., and Zuckerman, J.: Diagnostic examination of the eye. J. B. Lippincott Co., Philadelphia, 1946

Berliner, M. L.: Biomicroscopy of the eye. Hamish Hamilton Medical Books, London, 1949

Bier, N.: Contact lens routine and practice. Butterworths Scientific Publishers, London, 1957

Bier, N.: Paper read at New England Council of Optometrists Meeting, Boston, March 13-16, 1966

Black, C. J.: Ocular, anatomic, and physiologic changes due to contact lenses. Ill Med J 118:179-81, Nov 60

Boberg-Ans, J.: Experience in clinical examination of corneal sensitivity; corneal sensitivity and nasolarcrimal reflex after retrobulbular anaesthesia. Brit J Ophthal 39:705-26, Dec 55

Boyd, H. H.: Two-day adaptation to contact lenses. In Corneal and scleral lenses. Edited by L. J. Girard. C. V. Mosby Co., St. Louis, 1967

Bronson, N. R., II: Attachment of slit lamp photography. Trans Amer Acad Ophthal Otolaryng 70:858-60, Sep-Oct 66

Brucker, D., and Carter, D. B.: Corneal metabolism and contact lenses, chapter 8. Encyclopedia of Contact Lens Practice 2:42-66, 15 Jan 61

Brungardt, T. F.: Study of corneal contour measurements. Amer J Optom 39:596-602, Nov 62

Calmettes, L., et al.: Etude histologique et histochemique de l'epithelium anterieur de la cornee et da ses basales. Arch Ophthal 16:481-506, Jul-Aug 56

Cogan, D. G., and Kinsey, V. E.: Cornea. Physiological aspects. Arch Ophthal 28:661-9, Oct 42

Cohen, S.: Photography in optometric practice. Optom Weekly 57:54-6, 14 Jul 66

Daily, L., Jr., and Daily, R. K.: Modification of corneal contact lenses, vol. I. In International Ophthalmology Clinics. Little, Brown and Co., Boston, 1961

125

Davson, H.: The physiology of the eye. Ed. 2. Little, Brown and Co., Boston, 1963

Dickinson, F.: Some corneal changes associated with wearing of contact lenses. Brit J Physiol Opt 17:161-70, Jul 60

Dixon, J. M.: Ocular changes due to contact lenses. Amer J Ophthal 58:424-43, Sep 64

Dixon, J. M., Lawaczeck, E.: Corneal dimples and bubbles under corneal contact lenses. Amer J Ophthal 54:827-31, Nov 62

Doggart, J. H.: Ocular signs in slit-lamp microscopy. C. V. Mosby Co., St. Louis, 1949
  a. *Op. cit.*, p. 11
  b. *Op. cit.*, pp. 11-19

Duke-Elder, S., Ed.: System of Ophthalmology. C. V. Mosby Co., St. Louis, 1962, vol. 7

Duke-Elder, S., Ed.: System of Ophthalmology. C. V. Mosby Co., St. Louis, 1965, vol. 8

Farris, R. L., et al.: Corneal oxygen flux in contact lens wearers. In Corneal and scleral lenses. Edited by L. J. Girard. C. V. Mosby Co., St. Louis, 1967

Francois, J., and Rabaey, M.: The anatomy of the cornea. In The Transparency of the cornea. Edited by S. Duke-Elder and E. S. Perkins. Blackwell Scientific Publication, Oxford, 1960

Gambs Co.: Instruction book to photo slit 1000. Gambs Co., Lyon France

Girard, L. J.: Corneal contact lenses. C. V. Mosby Co., St. Louis, 1964

Goldberg, J. B.: Corneal curvature and refractive changes induced by corneal lenses observed immediately after removal and related to time. The Opt Weekly, Vol. 59, No. 15, Apr 1968, pp. 31-35

Goldberg, J. B.: Biomicroscopy photography. Unpublished paper read at the Contact Lens Section of the American Academy of Optometry, Columbus, December 13, 1964

Gordon, S.: Factors determining the physical and physiological fit of corneal type contact lenses. Some aspects of 'venting' in corneal contact lenses, chapter 6. Encyclopedia of Contact Lens Practice 2:6-34, 15 Jul 61

Goodlaw, E. I.: Use of slit lamp biomicroscopy in the fitting of contact lenses, chapter 11. Encyclopedia of Contact Lens Practice 3:5-43, 15 Nov 61

Grosvenor, T. P.: Physiological factors in contact lens wearing. The Optom Weekly, 57:13-19, Mar 31, 1966
  a. *Op. cit.*, p. 13-19

Haynes, P. R., Brungardt, T. F., and Pollock, E. D.: Use of fleuorescein in the fitting of contact lenses, chapter 10. Encyclopedia of Contact Lens Practice. 1 May 60, p. 11

Hill, R. M., and Fatt, I.:
  a. Oxygen measurements under a contact lens. Amer J Optom 41:382-7, Jun 64
  b. Deprivation of the cornea by contact lenses and lid closure. Amer J Optom 41:678-87, Nov 64

Hill, R. M., and Leighton, A. J.: Physiological time courses associated with contact lens temperature. I. Animal time courses with scleral lenses. Amer J Optom 30:427-38, Sep 63

Hill, R. M., and Leighton, A. J.: Physiological time courses associated with contact lens temperature. II. Animal time courses with scleral lenses. Amer J Optom 31:3-9, Feb 64

Hill, R. M., and Leighton, A. J.: Temperature changes of human cornea and tears under contact lenses.
  a. I. The relaxed open eye, and the natural and forced closed eye conditions. Amer J. Optom 42:9-16, Jan 65
  b. II. Effects of intermediate lid apertures and gaze. Amer J Optom 42:71-7, Feb 65

Hirano, J.: Histological studies on the corneal changes induced by corneal contact lenses. Jap J Ophthal 3:1-8, Jan-Mar 59

Jakus, M. A.: Studies on the cornea. II. The fine structure of Descemet's membrane. J Biophys Cytol 2:25, Jul 56

Jakus, M. A.: Ocular fine structure. Selected selectron micrographs. Little, Brown and Co., Boston, 1964

Johnson, L. V. and Erkhardt, R. E.: Rosacea keratitis and conditions with vascularization of the cornea treated with riboflavin. Arch. Ophth., 23:902, 1940

Jordan, H. E.: The textbook of histology. Appleton-Century-Crofts, Inc., New York, 1937

Kaps, S.: Optometrist, Tenafly, N. J., personal communication

Koby, F. E.: Slit-lamp microscopy of the living eye. Translated by C. Goulden and C. L. Harris. P. Blakiston's Sons and Co., Inc., Philadelphia, 1930
   a. *Op. cit.,* p. 36

Koetting, R. A.: Useful auxiliary tests in contact lens examination. Amer Optom Ass 36:439-42, Aug 65

Korb, D.: Recent advances in corneal lens fenestration, Appendix B. Encyclopedia of Contact Lens Practice 3:58-66, I Jan 62

Kraar, R. S., and Cummings, C. M.: Lacrimination, corneal sensitivity and corneal abrasive resistance in contact lens wearability. Optom Weekly 56:25-32, 18 Nov 65

La Tessa, et al.: Histochemistry of basement membrane of cornea. Amer J Ophthal 38:171-7, Aug 54

Lauber, H., In discussion on Deutsch, A.: Praktische Durchfuhrung von Myopiekorrektion mit Kontaktglasern. Klin. Monatsbl. Augenh., 82:535, 1929

Lester, R.: Fleuorscein and contact lenses. In Contacto. The National Research Foundation, Chicago, 1958.

Lester, R.: The use of the biomicroscope in contact lens fitting. The Optom. Weekly, 50:2261-2270, 1959.

Mandell, R. B.: Contact lens practice. Basic and advanced. Charles C. Thomas Publisher, Springfield, Ill., 1965

Maurice, D. M.: The permeability of the cornea. In the transparency of the cornea. Edited by S. Duke-Elder and F. S. Perkins. Blackwell Scientific Publications, Oxford, 1960

Maurice, D. M.: The cornea and sclerea, vol I. In the eye. Edited by H. Davson. Academic Press, New York, 1962

Mazow, B.: Personal communication

Neill, Sohnges, and Dickinson,: A second report on the fitting and use of microlenses. Amer J Opty, 31:8 (Aug. 1954) pp. 411-415

Neisel, P.: Spaltlampen photographie mit de hagg-streit-spaltlampe 900. Ophthalmologica(Basel) 151:489-504, 000 66

Norton, H. J.: Absolute stereophotography of the slit lamp optical section. A new ophthalmic stereograph. Amer J Ophthal 58:797-804, Nov 64

Ruben, M.: Recent developments in contact lens practice, vol. I. In the contact lens. Middlesex, England, 1:5-10, Oct 1967

Sampson, W. G.: Corneal edema. In Corneal and scleral contact lenses. Edited by L. J. Girard. C. V. Mosby Co., St. Louis, 1967

Schapero, M.: Tissue changes associated with contact lenses. Amer J Optom 43:477-99, Aug 66

Schirmer, K. E.: Corneal sensitivity and contact lenses. Brit J Ophthal 47:493-5, Aug 63

Schirmer, K. E.: Microfilm photography in ophthalmology. Brit J Ophthal 49:76-9, Feb 65

Schirmer, K. E., and Mellor, L. D.: Corneal sensitivity after cataract extraction. Arch Ophthal (Chicago) 65:433-6, Mar 61

Smelser, G. K.: Relation of factors involved in maintenance of optical properties of cornea to contact lens wear. AMA Arch Ophthal (Chicago) 47:328-43, Mar 52

Smelser, G. K., and Chen, D. K.: Physiological changes in cornea induced by contact lenses. AMA Arch Ophthal (Chicago) 53:676-9, Mar 55

Smelser, G. K., and Ozanics, V. I.: Importance of atmospheric oxygen for maintenance of the optical properties of the human cornea. Science 115:140, 1 Feb 52

Strebel, J.: Objective proof for the orthopedic effect of contact lenses on keratoconus. Klin Mbl Augenheilk 99:30-5, Jul 37

Strughold, H.: The Sensitivity of cornea and conjuctiva of the hyman eye and the use of contact lenses. Amer J Optom 30:625-30, Dec 53

Thomas, G. I.: The Cornea. Charles C. Thomas Publishers, Springfield, Ill., 1955

Index

129

Appendix

ERRATA AND ADDITIONAL DATA

As it is with publishing, tiny errors creep into the pages, and late additions are frequently inserted to give readers the benefit of new data after the book is printed. The following changes and additions fall in these categories. Several full pages are also reproduced correctly.

Color plates A-11 and B-19: The caption for Figure A-11 should be listed under Figure B-19. The caption for Figure B-19 should be listed under Figure A-11.

Page 23: Figure II-18 should appear as shown below.

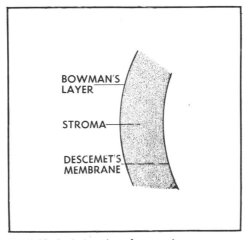

Fig. II-18. Optical section of a normal cornea

Pages 96 and 97: The reference (Figure V-5) on Page 96 should appear on Page 97 at the end of the first paragraph.

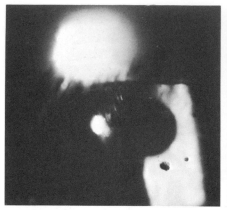
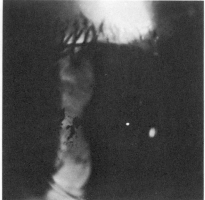

Fig. II-28 (left). Pigment deposits on posterior corneal surface of aphakic patient, retro-illumination.
Fig. II-29 (right). Foreign material on the front surface of a corneal lens seen with retro-illumination, high magnification.

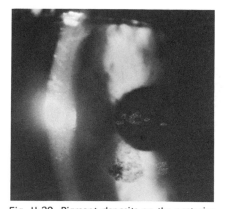

Fig. II-30. Pigment deposits on the posterior corneal surface of an aphakic patient. (The pigment deposits which are seen in light immediately reflected from the iris are exposed by retro-illumination; those on the adjacent, darker areas are seen in indirect illumination.)

between a dark pupil background and the central corneal clouding is enhanced when the pupil is dilated (Sampson, 1967).

While the overall size of the affected corneal area may be related to the overall contact lens size and its optic (central) zone diameter, Korb and Exford reported that the size of the affected area, in itself, is not an indication of the severity of the condition or of the probability of a subsequent abrasion.

Although central circular corneal clouding may be observed with the lens in situ, I prefer to investigate its severity when the lens is removed. Therefore,

29

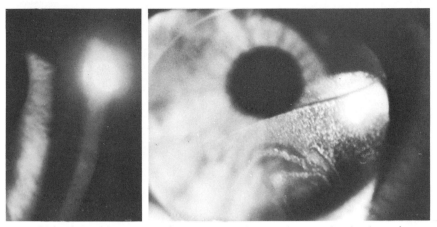

Fig. II-33 (left). Specular reflection. (The image from the posterior corneal surface is seen.)
Fig. II-34 (right). Poor wetting of corneal lens surface. Specular reflection, high magnification.

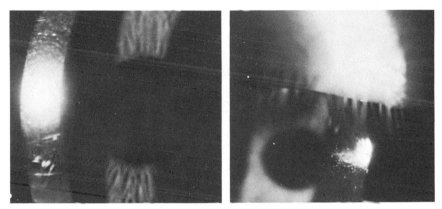

Fig. II-35 (left). Specular reflection exposes scratches on the front surface of a corneal lens, poor wetting characteristics of the front surface of the lens, and mucous formation on the lower part of the lens.
Fig. II-36 (right). Lacrimal debris seen with specular reflection, high magnification.

of a contact lens, is examined in the zone of specular reflection. The areas of the corneal endothelium observed when the incident light is temporally directed are different from those seen with nasally directed light.

Examination in the zone of specular reflection may expose small, posterior surface precipitates. These appear as black dots which mar the endothelial mosaic as do defects in the silvered surface of a mirror (Figs. II-33,34,35,36). This type of illumination is a very delicate method used to observe mucus and cell debris in the tears; to detect and assess changes on the anterior and posterior corneal surfaces; to study the endothelial cells, the anterior and posterior surfaces of the crystalline lens, the shagreen effect, and the epithelial cells of the

33

CORRECTED

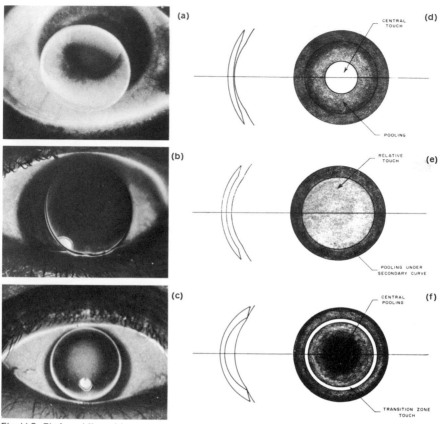

Fig. V-2. Fitting philosophies

Figs. V-2(a) and (b) (top). Apical bearing (photograph in 2(a) courtesy Solex Laboratories, Inc.).

Figs. V-2(c) and (d) (middle). Apical alignment.

Figs. V-2(e) and (f) (bottom). Apical clearance.

Historically, Touhy originally used the monocurve lens design (patented in 1950) to fit corneal contact lenses. This design was later modified by Neill, Sohnges, and Dickinson (1954). Touhy had made the contact lens base curve flatter than the flattest primary corneal meridian by 1.50 D. or more so that the curve formed is considered obsolete, although a modified version is used to fit corneal lenses in cases of keratoconus.

The original clinical use of the philosophy relied upon an appreciably flat, single ocular surface curve for peripheral corneal clearance. With apical bearing, the lens rests on the central cornea, has peripheral corneal clearance, and is rocked back and forth during blinking. According to Mandell (1965), the cornea has limited tolerance to the constant apical bearing. Since the lens movement often abrades the central cornea, wearing becomes uncomfortable and the lens is

CORRECTED

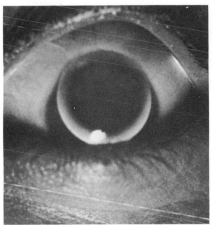 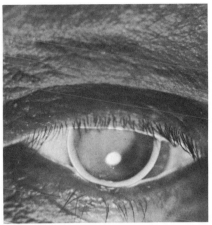

Fig. V-10 (left) and Fig. V-11 (right). Corneal lens fitted too securely peripherally.

may be retained, for example, for plus power lenses.

Lens Fit Too Secure Peripherally

A lens fit that is too secure peripherally is usually a *high-riding* lens in that part of the lens covers the cornea while another part impinges on the superior limbus or encroaches on the superior sclera. The cause is one of the following: (1) the overall lens size is too large; (2) the peripheral curve or curves are too wide and/or too flat, with the result that excessive edge standaway causes the lens to be displaced upward by the blink. When this occurs, it is likely that the optic zone diameter is too small (Figs. V-10,11).

Clinical Findings

The lens is fixed in position high on the cornea. There is insufficient peripheral clearance in those areas where the lens impinges on the superior limbus. This frequently causes the limbal vessels to fill and proliferate into the peripheral corneal areas. Occasionally, there is also conjunctival injection.

The high lens position is characteristic of an "on K" fit for corneal astigmatism of 2.00 D. or more (spherical base curve lens), especially for a lens of high minus power. Mandell (1965) stated that the cornea can easily support the lens in a high position because the center of gravity tends toward the posterior side of the lens. When the lens position is high the optic zone diameter often encroaches on the lower pupil areas and the patient may report visual distress concomitant with monocular diplopia.

With fluorescein and black light one observes deep lacrimal pooling in the superior quadrants; there is usually an absence of fluorescence in the areas of insufficient peripheral clearance. There is deep, continuous peripheral clearance beneath the inferior lens edges, especially when the lens stands away from the cornea.

104

CORRECTED

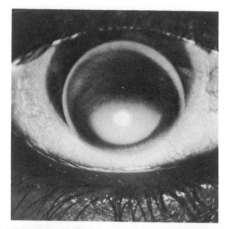

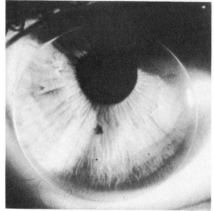

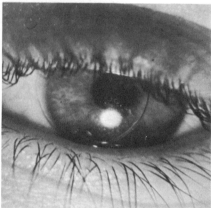

Fig. V-13 (top). Lens fitted too loose peripherally.
Fig. V-14 (left). A corneal lens fitted too loose peripherally; diffuse illumination, low magnification.
Fig. V-15 (right). Nasal displacement of corneal lens fitted too loose peripherally.

corneal asymmetry, particularly decentration of the corneal apex and non-uniform corneal flattening.

Clinical Findings

The lens does not center well. The displacement may be nasal or temporal, high or low. The peripheral areas often encroach on the pupil and induce visual disturbance. Often, the lens moves during blinking. Excessive lens movement may cause superficial epithelial disturbances such as punctates, stippling, and irregular linear staining. Occasionally, discomfort and visual distress result when mucous and lipid deposits form on the lens surfaces. Conjunctival injection may develop after relatively short periods of contact lens wear. The peri-limbal vessels

107

CORRECTED

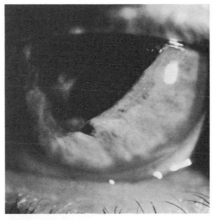

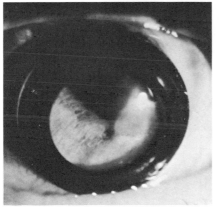 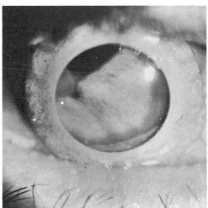

Fig. VI-4 (top). Sphincterotomy and scar tissue.
Fig. VI-5 (left). Opaque periphery corneal lens fitted for initial clinical investigation.
Fig. VI-6 (right). Early stages of fitting a cosmetic corneal lens.
Photographic history of cosmetic corneal lens fitting for sphincterotomy.

other instruments manufactured by the Zeiss Company. There is an anterior
segment illuminator which is a pilot light used to locate the position of the light
reflex and the electronic flash on the cornea so that the reflex will not appear in
the picture or obscure the condition to be photographed; this illuminator is
regulated for brightness by a recess disc with different apertures at the light exit.
The flash generator and transformer is a highly developed electronic apparatus
which supplies energy for the bulb and flash tube in the slit illuminator, the bulb
and flash tube in the anterior segment illuminator, and the bulb in the fixation
device. Stereo pictures may be taken when the small beam splitter is interposed
between the body of the microscope and the binocular tube. However, this
technique is not recommended because it produces a 50% loss of light, and the

116

CORRECTED